*ask*
# DR. KEITH

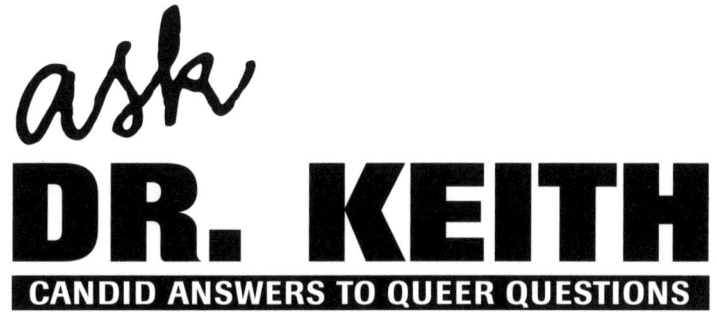

DR. KEITH LOUKES

whitecap

Copyright © 2004 by Dr. Keith Loukes
Whitecap Books

All rights reserved. No part of this publication may be reproduced, stored in a retrieval system, or transmitted in any form or by any means, electronic, mechanical, photocopying, recording or otherwise, without prior written permission of the publisher. All recommendations are made without guarantee on the part of the author or Whitecap Books Ltd. The author and publisher disclaim any liability in connection with the use of this information. For additional information, please contact Whitecap Books, 351 Lynn Avenue, North Vancouver, British Columbia, Canada V7J 2C4.
Visit our website at www.whitecap.ca

Edited by Barbara Pulling
Proofread by Lesley Cameron
Cover and interior design by Jacqui Thomas
Cover photography by Nathan Briggs

Printed and bound in Canada

LIBRARY AND ARCHIVES CANADA CATALOGUING IN PUBLICATION

Loukes, Keith, 1974-
    Ask Dr. Keith : candid answers to queer questions / Keith Loukes.

Includes bibliographical references and index.
ISBN 1-55285-607-0

    1. Gays—Sexual behavior. 2. Interpersonal relations. 3. Gays—Health and hygiene. I. Title.

HQ76.25.L68 2004     306.76'6     C2004-904148-7

The publisher acknowledges the financial support of the Government of Canada through the Book Publishing Industry Development Program for our publishing activities.

# Contents

| | | |
|---|---|---|
| | Introduction | 6 |
| **Chapter 1** | For Starters<br>Crushes, coming out, monogamy, masturbation, and more | 9 |
| **Chapter 2** | Ins and Outs<br>Anal sex, oral sex—<br>all kinds of penetration | 25 |
| | *A Queer Quiz* | 43 |
| **Chapter 3** | Girl Parts<br>Oral sex, dildos, clits, and more | 47 |
| **Chapter 4** | Boy Parts<br>"What is this?" and "where did it go?"<br>to "measuring up" and "getting it up" | 57 |
| | *You like WHAT?* | 78 |
| **Chapter 5** | Sexy & Safe: For the boys<br>When your plumbing acts up | 79 |
| **Chapter 6** | Sexy & Safe: For the girls<br>Why does it burn? Why do I itch? | 97 |
| | *What's bugging you?* | 114 |
| **Chapter 7** | What's Love Got to Do with It?<br>Questions about relationships | 115 |
| | Sources & Acknowledgements | 130 |
| | Index | 132 |
| | About the Author | 136 |

# Introduction

SEXUALITY HAS ALWAYS BEEN A HOT TOPIC, but until the latter half of the twentieth century, discussion about it was mostly confined to the bedroom. The North American hetero world came bursting through the bedroom door after the repressive 1950s with the "sexual revolution." People became increasingly comfortable with discussing and expressing their sexuality; and this talk soon spread to more public forums. Column after column of sex and relationship advice started to appear in magazines and newspapers. Cinema began to open up sexually as well, with films that previously would have been judged too racy to be screened. North American TV, although it still lags behind its European counterpart, has recently begun to catch up.

However, most of this advancement in public sexual discourse has been targeted at straight men and women. Homosexuality and bisexuality, despite being part of the sexual revolution and gaining in acceptability ever since, are still neglected in a culture where heterosexuality is seen as the norm. Until recently, transgendered people were barely recognized, and they still face heavy cultural stigmatization. Generally speaking, those of us who don't identify as straight face limits on where we can openly discuss our sexuality, due to a common public disregard (and often disgust) towards the way in which we practise it. Many gay, lesbian, bisexual, and transgendered (GLBT) folks have no one to talk to, personally or professionally, because of the deep shadows of the closet in which some of us are still forced to live. Thankfully, we are finding new opportunities to talk, inquire, and exchange experiences. Today we see sex columns in numerous queer publications, queer life depicted in the theatre, and gay- and lesbian-oriented television programming.

I stand in this newly developing arena. I've been answering people's sex and relationship questions on the air at Pridevision TV (the first 24/7 GLBT television station in the world) since January 2001. I feel pretty comfortable doing so, since I have a medical background and some experience in counselling. (Although I'm not a "sexpert," as some people have called me in the past.) The questions I receive range from the straightforward (should I be using the word "straight" here?) to the, er, more unusual. Whatever the case, there is an insatiable hunger in the GLBT community for talking about these issues in a positive environment.

You might notice a lack of transgender content. Although I've included one or two questions touching on this issue, I cannot do it justice in this book. I hope to explore transgenderism in more detail in another forum in the future.

My deepest thanks to those who have submitted questions over the past few years. Without you, this book would not exist. Although I've often combined two or more questions for the purposes of the book, and changed many names, some of you may recognize yourself in these pages. I've tried to include a broad array of questions, touching on as many issues as possible. However, this is not a reference text. Nor is it meant to replace professional advice from your doctor or therapist. Nothing can ever replace an interactive, properly focussed discussion of your specific concerns. But being able to pose questions in a "Dear Abby" format does allow people to ask things they might be shy about discussing in person. I hope you'll find my book both entertaining and playfully educational.

So, dive in and enjoy. I encourage all of you to keep asking questions. Ask your friends. Ask your doctor. Ask me. It's only through this kind of discussion that we'll gain a better understanding of ourselves and each other.

Until next time, I wish you health and happiness.

Dr. Keith Loukes

# 1

# For Starters

Crushes, coming out, monogamy, masturbation, and more

❝ **Dear Dr. Keith,**

I am a 16-year-old gay male. I have known I'm gay for a long time. But I live in a small town, and I feel as though I can't tell anyone. No one would understand. I don't know anybody else who is gay, either. I have a secret crush on my best friend, but he has a girlfriend. I feel really bad about this. Can you help? ❞

Tim

Dear Tim,

Having a crush on your best friend while you're growing up seems to be a time-honoured tradition in the gay world—a rite of passage experienced by many. Sometimes it has a happy ending, but more often than not it ends in heartache. Does this make it any easier, knowing that you are far from alone in having secret feelings for someone you're close to? Likely not.

With regards to your feelings for your friend, it's a tough call. Divulging your interest in him is a gamble. Although it's possible he may respond in kind, it is more likely that he may not be able to return those feelings. He might understand, shrug it off, and appreciate your being honest. Or he may start to feel uncomfortable around you, changing your friendship. On the flip side, not telling him how you feel could eat at you so much it destroys the friendship in the process. This is the dilemma you face.

There is another possibility, though. How about redirecting your feelings to someone who will be receptive to them? Living in a small town can be a huge barrier. There are proportionally fewer people around. Add to this a possible fear of being labelled and/or made an outcast by the community, and it means that other gay people are simply more difficult to find.

Fortunately, the addition of the Internet to the dating world has managed to connect people in smaller towns who feel strongly about not outing themselves. It's an easy way to meet others similar to yourself, allowing you to build a network of friends and potential relationships. So get connected if you can, and meet some people you can relate to on-line. A word of caution, however—protect yourself by never giving out personal information or agreeing to meet strangers except in public places.

The Internet is also a great source of on-line support and information about being gay. See the Sources & Acknowledgements section at the back of this book for some ideas on where to start.

Only you can decide whether the gamble of telling your friend is worth it, or if you should leave things as they are and wait for your feelings to fade. (They will, trust me.) My guess is that finding someone else to be the target of your love will make you much happier either way.

**" Dear Dr. Keith,**

**Can a person change his or her sexual orientation? "**

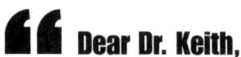

**David**

Dear David,

There *are* homophobic people who think that you can change your sexual orientation. There are camps throughout North America, most of them religion-based, which profess to "treat" homosexuality as if it were a mental illness. These conversion camps use various methods of persuasion and mountains of anti-gay propaganda to try to convince gay, lesbian, bisexual, and transgendered people that they are ill and can choose to be heterosexual. It's brainwashing, pure and simple.

Talk to individuals who claim to be "cured," i.e., no longer queer, and all you'll get is a response programmed into their heads by someone else. It is well accepted in medical, psychological, and sociological circles that orientation cannot be changed. "Converted" queers must live with a constant internal struggle that destabilizes their psychological state. I feel sorry for these people who, in seeking "treatment," are actually hurting themselves further.

You are what you are. You can't change the fundamental things that make you the person you are, including your sexual orientation. You can change what's on the surface, but the heart of you remains deep inside. Accepting that is accepting yourself—and that can't fail to lead you to good things.

## " Dear Dr. Keith,

**Why do some people use the term "LGBT" while others say "GLBT"? And what does "LGBTTQ" mean?** "

Paulo

Dear Paulo,

GLBT and LGBT (the letters, in whichever order, stand for gay, lesbian, bisexual, and transgendered) are used interchangeably. Why the position of the "G" and the "L" is sometimes switched, I'm not really sure—perhaps to avoid favouring one group over the other.

The additional letters in the term LGBTTQ refer to two-spirited people (the aboriginal term for queer people, which encompasses those who are transgendered) and to people who are *queer* or *questioning*. I have often seen an "I" added into the mix as well, to include people who are *intersexed*, or hermaphrodites—born with both male and female physical traits.

I think the time has come to just call us "NYAH": not your average heterosexual. Anyone out there agree with me?

## ❝ Dear Dr. Keith,

**I'm really upset with my family. They are uncomfortable with me being gay, and they don't want anyone else to know. It always hurts to be excluded from a family gathering, and I have problems accepting that this is to be my fate due to my "chosen lifestyle." I feel like I am being forced to choose between my family and my partner. Help!** ❞

**Alicia**

Dear Alicia,

It's sad to hear stories about people at odds with their families over their sexual orientation, but unfortunately it's a bleak reality. Although GLBT rights are furthered every day, there always seem to be people who refuse to let us just live and be happy. Some people deal with their homophobia by not dealing with it at all. They avoid situations where they might have to confront it, like family events. Excluding a GLBT member from family gatherings is a cowardly way of "sweeping dirt under the rug." You don't have to choose. Your family does. Sit down with the major offenders, and explain both how much you care for them and how much their behaviour is hurting you. Tell them that it's not fair for you and your partner to be excluded, and that if they truly care for you in return, they will welcome the two of you at family functions. If they still refuse to acknowledge you and your partner, their choice has been made. They are turning their backs on you, not vice versa. Their position might soften over time—who knows? But you have done all you can.

There's no question that it's hard to be rejected by your family. But if it comes down to that, stick to your guns. Choose your partner, and your lifestyle, over your family's homophobia. Hopefully, over time, they'll see that shunning you was a mistake.

> **Dear Dr. Keith,**
>
> **I have a gay friend who is addicted to going out and picking up men. It used to happen every few weeks, but I have just found out that he is out drinking and cruising for guys at least once a week. His other friends and I are considering having an intervention to tell him that we are worried about his health and his obsession with sex. He has recently come out of the closet, and I know that sometimes men have to go through this period. But when does it become a problem? Should we intervene or leave him to "sow his wild oats"?**
>
> **Shawn**

Dear Shawn,

Your friend is lucky to have a group of people so concerned about him.

Coming out can be a very liberating experience. There can also be a natural tendency to overcompensate for the years of alienation and being alone by surrounding yourself with many partners. To a degree, this is normal, providing the person is not adversely affecting his job, health, or other relationships. I know quite a few well-balanced guys who go to bars and "pick up" on a weekly basis.

My advice is to let your friend do his thing. If you see serious problems arising at any point, an "intervention" might be in order. In that case, you should sit your friend down, explain why you are concerned, and remain very supportive. Since people in this kind of situation may perceive their friends as being overly critical, tread carefully. But as long as your friend truly understands how you feel about him, and why you are concerned, it should be okay.

> **Dear Dr. Keith,**
>
> **How important is monogamy in a gay relationship? Is it different for male-male and female-female relationships?**
>
> **John**

Dear John,

The great thing about people is that we are all different. Some people prefer snacking on chocolate rather than peanuts. Some would rather wear blue shirts than green. Some prefer playing music to playing sports. And some of us prefer a monogamous relationship over a relationship that includes outside sexual partners. There is no question, though, that differing opinions about the importance of monogamy inside a relationship can be disastrous unless addressed carefully. Obviously, when two people prefer monogamy and honour that, there is little problem. But when one or both like to have sex outside of the relationship, accusations of cheating can arise and cause great upset. Non-monogamy should be discussed carefully and agreed upon by both partners before such an event occurs.

There are happy couples everywhere on both sides of the debate, male and female alike. Gay men may be more likely than lesbians to prefer sleeping around to sleeping with only one partner; stereotypes certainly suggest that. Regardless of gender, though, monogamy is not necessary to create a successful relationship. What *is* necessary is an agreement that's understood by both partners.

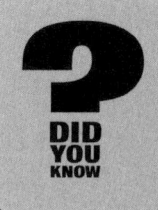

**DID YOU KNOW** The Greek letter "lambda" was chosen by the Gay Activists Alliance in New York City in 1970 to become their symbol for gay equality. The rainbow flag, which represents GLBT pride, was designed by Gilbert Baker of San Francisco in 1978 and was quickly adopted worldwide.

**❝ Dear Dr. Keith,**

**The guy I'm interested in says he's straight, but he acts another way. (Hint, hint.) What should I do: go by what he says or what he does? ❞**

**Tommy**

Dear Tommy,

Go by what he says.

I assume by "hint, hint" you mean you and he are fooling around. Some straight guys do this. So there really could be no more he is able to offer you.

But whether or not this guy is straight has nothing to do

with why I'd advise you to walk away from this. The important thing here is that he's *telling* you he's straight, and therefore, in so many words, that he isn't interested in pursuing a relationship. He might change his mind in the future, but for now you won't be doing yourself much good by sticking around and hoping that he switches.

Why not find yourself someone who wants to give you more? You'll be much happier in the end.

**❝ Dear Dr. Keith,**

**I don't understand the difference between being "transgendered" and "transsexual," and I see these words used around the community all the time. Please explain! ❞**

**Nadia**

Dear Nadia,

I don't blame you for being confused. I sometimes have to stop and think about these words myself. Transgenderism is an umbrella term that refers to a person's thinking and/or behaviour crossing traditional gender lines. This can include the way the person acts, dresses, talks, identifies, etc.

A transsexual (trannie) is a transgendered person who believes their biological gender (i.e., their gender at birth) does not match the gender they identify with. Transsexuals, often, but not always, will seek surgery to alter their bodies to the desired gender.

Someone whose gender identity does match their biological gender, yet who prefers to wear the opposite gender's clothing, is called a transvestite (cross-dresser). An example of this is men who wear female clothing for enjoyment but still see themselves as male ("drag queens" usually fall into this category). As you can see, the key difference between the two ways of identifying comes from the person's perception of their psychological gender.

> **Dear Dr. Keith,**
>
> **I have known that I'm bisexual for at least three years. I don't find it difficult approaching either women or men, but I also want to be in a stable relationship. It seems as though this will never happen, although I have had many affairs. What am I doing wrong?**
>
> **Moira**

Dear Moira,

It sounds as if you're saying that, despite your ability to approach potential partners, you're having difficulty creating something more permanent than a "fling."

Your question is not an easy one to answer. What exactly are you looking for? At its most basic, a long-term relationship boils down to an understanding between two people with comparable expectations. Relationships have two broad components: the physical and the emotional. Often a relationship will be a mixture of the two, but sometimes it can be solely one or the other.

The physical side is the attraction, the desire, the sexual activity. The emotional side encompasses your feelings and your needs to share, communicate, explore, and be involved with each another in non-sexual ways. Both people come to a new relationship with their own preference about how much "physical" and how much "emotional" they want the relationship to contain, thus creating their own "recipes" for an ideal partnership. When these recipes of expectations differ too much, problems between the two people arise.

For example, if one person wants less "physical" and more "emotional" while the other is looking only for the "physical," expectations clash, and the relationship likely ends in failure. However, if both people's recipes agree, then the relationship has the potential to be successful.

Moira, your recipe sounds as if it calls for more emotional ingredients, with less importance placed on the physical ones. So you need to find someone who "cooks with the same book." Lay your expectations out tactfully with potential partners at the beginning, so they are clear about what you are looking for. With luck, Mr. or Ms. Right will soon come along.

Oh, and sorry about the cooking analogy. I really should stick to practising medicine!

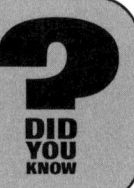

In 2003, Canada became one of only three countries in the world where people have the right to marry someone of the same sex. The other two are Belgium and the Netherlands. As it stands, the future of this right is anything but certain…

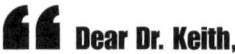  Dear Dr. Keith,

I'm a 22-year-old gay man. I've been living in a big city for twelve years but have never had a relationship with another gay man. I've tried going to different gay communities in the city, but I'm not accepted as who I am. I believe this is because of my feminine side. Other gay people don't want to have me as their friend or partner because I'm a sissy guy.

I'm a blond, blue-eyed cute boy, and people are usually impressed with how I look. But they don't show any more reaction than that. Do you think there are guys out there who are interested in having a long-term relationship with a sissy guy? I just find myself so helpless.

Jamie

Dear Jamie,

A feminine gay man is not a rare commodity in the gay community. There are feminine-acting straight guys, too. Everyone is different, especially in how "masculine" they come across. It certainly casts no reflection on who you are as a person. I myself prefer to see someone a little feminine to men who overact the porn-star "butch" bit. To me, that's totally unappealing.

Just as there are many different levels of femininity and masculinity, there are many different levels of preference. You often notice guys in ads proclaiming themselves as "straight-acting, seeking same." But are there also guys out there who seek "screaming queens"? Absolutely. Just as some guys prefer blonds or men with a bit of facial hair, others have a strong predilection for guys who are considered less than butch.

Be proud of who you are, and don't try to hide it. If you're "nelly," then learn to love it. It's only a negative feature if you portray it that way. It's yours; it's you. It colours your personality and will make you adorable to a lot of people. (Look at Jack from *Will & Grace*. What's not to love?) Anyone who dismisses you because they think you're too feminine doesn't deserve someone as great as you. Right? So go find yourself a nelly-lover—they really do exist.

**❝ Dear Dr. Keith,**

**My friends say I'm good-looking. How come I can't get laid?**

**Kevin**

Dear Kevin,

If you just want to "get laid," there are many avenues you can pursue. Bars aren't the only place to meet guys for sex. Every city has its own cruising area, usually a park or a remote parking lot. In large cities there are bathhouses or saunas where you pay money to enter a private establishment, take off your clothes, find someone you like, and let testosterone do the rest. There are also many on-line "looking for sex" sites you can try. (Keep in mind that with all of these options there is some risk to your health and safety, so be careful.)

However—and call me old-fashioned—I think the best sex is with someone you know well and have feelings for. Get out there, meet people through friends, approach people in bars, look on-line, date actively. Find someone you like and who likes you back. That's good sex.

I sense some self-esteem issues here. Just as dogs can smell fear, homos can definitely smell poor self-image. So my best advice to you is this: (1) Be confident in who you are. You are attractive. (Would your friends lie?) (2) Don't forget to wear condoms when having sex. The last thing you need to boost your confidence is to "get laid," then "get infections." Cheers!

**❝ Dear Dr. Keith,**

**Can a person really go blind from masturbating too much?**

**Vinny**

Dear Vinny,

No, of course not. This myth was likely generated long ago by those who felt that masturbation was "bad" and wanted to discourage people from doing it. It is in reality a very acceptable and healthy practice. It leads to an enhanced knowledge of your body and of ways to produce pleasure. Plus, if you're gay, it gives you experience using the equipment, right? Go for it!

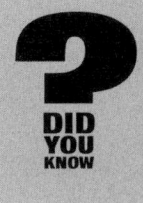

Homosexuality was diagnosed as an illness until the latter part of the twentieth century. It was not removed from the standard psychiatry text, *The Diagnostic and Statistical Manual of Mental Disorders* (*DSM*, for short), until 1973.

# 2
# Ins and Outs

Anal sex, oral sex—all kinds of penetration

**THE RECORD FOR THE MOST ORGASMS** recorded in one hour is 134 for a woman, and 16 for a man.

❝ **Dear Dr. Keith,**

**I've never been a bottom, but now I'm with a guy who's a top, and he wants me to bottom for him. What do I do to prepare?**

**Also, about douching. Do I need to do this after we have sex? If so, what brand should I use? I know there are douches made for women, but is there one for guys as well?** ❞

**Joe**

Dear Joe,

Patience is the key to being a bottom. It takes a lot of relaxation and getting used to the sensation in order to receive anal intercourse. The more tense and apprehensive you are, the more you will feel the urge to "bear down," making penetration more difficult. I always recommend that guys experiment with fingers or small toys at first (alone, or with your partner). Using lots of lubrication, gradually increase the objects in size until you think you are ready to take something the size of your partner's penis.

Anal douching is a common practice for gay men who bottom, usually coming from the desire to be "clean" and also to prevent any "mess" that may result from anal penetration. Men commonly use a variety of products for this, from female douching products to enemas (insertion of water into the colon by tubing).

Douching is certainly not necessary before or after anal sex, and many couples don't bother. In fact, I am wary of it. Frequent douching can lead to constipation, and in severe situations chronic enemas become necessary in order to move your bowels. In addition to this, there is some medical evidence that douching can sufficiently irritate the lining of your rectum to increase the risk of HIV transmission. The prepared female products should be avoided, since they often contain scents and other chemicals designed to make a woman feel more "fresh." In fact, many gynecologists recommend that women avoid them as well.

If you want to clean up beforehand, I recommend using an ear syringe (a rubber bulb with a small spout on the end, obtainable at most pharmacies for under $10). Lubricate the tip well and insert into the rectum, rinsing several times before sex. The small amount of water used is less irritating and less likely to cause long-term problems.

Happy humping!

**❝ Dear Dr. Keith,**

**I was wondering if taking a muscle relaxant would help reduce the pain of anal sex. ❞**

**Vanilla Boy**

Dear Vanilla Boy,

Pain during anal sex can often be a warning sign that something "down there" isn't right. Or sometimes the anus may just be too tight to allow penetration.

It's questionable that muscle relaxants would help if tightness is the issue. Using them may make you drowsy and might put you to sleep. (So why bother?) On top of this, over-the-counter relaxants are not of much use in relaxing muscles, despite the ads you see on television. So I don't think they will be of much benefit in the long run.

Some people use alcohol to "loosen up" before sex (pun intended). A drink or two may help you to relax, allowing your partner to penetrate you more easily. However, you don't want your sex life to depend on alcohol. In addition, should you drink too much, you may receive an injury that you are not aware of until it's too late. Also factor in that excessive alcohol use can impair your judgement around safe sex practices.

My advice to you is this: go to your doctor and get an examination to rule out anything that might be causing pain in your rectum. Then start anal play with your partner, using *lots* and *lots* of lubrication, inserting small things like fingers to begin with. Build up gradually to larger items, using discomfort as your guide: if it hurts, stop and try something smaller again. Eventually you will train your body to be able to take larger items, including your partner's penis.

Bottoms up!

**" Dear Dr. Keith,**

**I am new to anal sex, and I love it. In fact, I use toys I bought online to practise. Every time I use them, however, some shit comes out. This is totally gross, and I am afraid that I will shit all over my new boyfriend. (We haven't had sex yet; I am too scared.) Help me quick! "**

**Zack**

Dear Zack,

What you are describing is completely normal in every way—part of the experience that makes up anal sex. It always has been and always will be messy. That can't be avoided. (In fact, I think that's why towels were invented.)

If you want to minimize the mess, go to the toilet before sex, then gently clean the anus and rectum with soap and water. Alternatively, you can rinse inside with a bit of water. (See my advice to Joe on page 27 for more information on that.)

Remember I mentioned towels? Lay one down on the mattress before you start, to save yourself from having to wash your sheets after every trip to bed. Have fun!

---

The largest penis in the animal kingdom belongs to the mighty blue whale. This animal provides no less than 11 feet (3.35 m) of fully functional hot whale action.

The largest vagina in the animal kingdom belongs to the female blue whale. On average, it is between 6 and 8 feet (1.8 and 2.4 m) in depth.

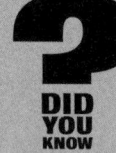

**DID YOU KNOW**

---

**❝ Dear Dr. Keith:**

**I recently joined an Internet dating service, and I have met guys on there who want me to fuck them bare. I know this is risky behaviour, and I would just as soon play safe, but isn't the bottom in more danger than the top for the risk of infections and disease (HIV)? Why are men wanting this when they know it is dangerous? Please help explain the risks to the giver (top man), me, if I do this for them. ❞**

**Gordon**

Dear Gordon,

In a recent study, 14 per cent of almost 400 men who sleep with men reported barebacking—defined in the study as having intentional unprotected sex with a non-primary partner—in the past two years. More than a third of these men had sex with someone of a different or unknown HIV status.

This rising trend is a huge topic of concern. Some say that the community doesn't fear contracting HIV disease like they used to, as they perceive HIV infection to be "not a big deal" with all of the treatments we have available. Others hypothesize that the abundance of public education out there has encouraged thrill-seekers to "live on the edge."

Back to your question: is barebacking riskier for the bottom? Absolutely. The top's risk is less, since the skin in the anus and rectum are more fragile than the skin on the penis. However, the risk to the top is still significant, because it only takes one small nick or scratch on the top's genitals for the virus to be transmitted.

You're gambling when you bareback, especially with strangers. My advice to you is that your health is worth more than what some consider an exciting and risky romp in the sheets. So—always wrap it up.


**❝ Dear Dr. Keith,**

**Someone once told me the inside of the rectum is as fragile as a wet tissue. If this is true, then why don't I hemorrhage when I am fisted? ❞**

**Gregory**


Dear Gregory,

Comparing the rectum to a wet tissue is a bit of an overexaggeration. The lining of the rectum is actually quite resistant and tough; it has to be, in order to withstand the abuse its purpose demands of it—the passage of stool. Your rectum and lower bowel are basically a hose-shaped layer of special membrane that absorbs water from what you have eaten. This membrane or mucosa is surrounded by layers of muscle that propel the waste through, making for a relatively sturdy structure.

That being said, there is always such a thing as too much force leading to injury, resulting in tearing and bleeding unless a certain level of caution is observed. Before taking anything into your rectum, make sure that your rectum is big enough to stretch around that object; otherwise, you could be in trouble. The ability to take a fist safely doesn't happen overnight. For most people, it takes months to years of gentle stretching to be able to accommodate something as large in diameter as a fist.

**❝ Dear Dr. Keith,**

**My boyfriend and I have been together for over four years. We are still using condoms, and maybe always will, but that is not my question. We want to take our relationship a little further, and we would like to know the proper procedure for me to start being able to take my partner's fist. We know that I must be thoroughly cleaned out first, and then use lots of lube and, most importantly, go slowly and relax. Do you have any other suggestions? ❞**

**Larry**

Dear Larry,

Questions about fisting are often shrouded in embarrassment and fear of judgement from others. It may not be everyone's cup of tea, but the stigma attached to this practice is unfortunate. Fisting must be done with extreme care, but if it's done safely, it can be enjoyable for both partners.

The anus is made up of two rings of muscle called sphincters, which are lined by a special skin-like layer called mucosa. Except during bowel movements, these muscle rings are normally contracted. While muscles are generally rubbery and pliable, they do have limits as to how much they can be stretched in a short period of time. If you stretch the sphincters too quickly, you could injure them or their overlying lining, causing tears, inflammation, local infections, or even rupture of the bowel wall.

However, muscles can be conditioned to be more accommodating by gentle, repeated stretching over time (this is how dancers stretch their legs to improve flexibility, for example). In the case of anal penetration, this can be accomplished by slowly increasing the size of the penetrating object over time, starting with fingers and small toys. Use pain as your guide: if it hurts, STOP. Only when you're able to allow the penetration of a toy the diameter of a fist are you ready for fisting.

Here are some fisting rules:

(1) You may wish to cleanse your bowel before anal play. While this is probably not necessary, it may reduce the complications of infection, if injury to the bowel lining were to occur. Anything used to penetrate (fingers, fists, arms) should be cleaned well first, and covered in latex.

(2) Lubrication is key. There is no such thing as too much lubrication, but too little can cause huge problems.

(3) The receiving partner must relax, allowing the penetrator to stretch the outer muscle, then the inner muscle, slowly. This takes at least a few minutes, probably more. After the fist is comfortably inside, a slow in-and-out movement can be tried.

(4) Pain is not normal. Neither is bleeding. If you experience either, STOP IMMEDIATELY.

Be safe, and enjoy!

> **Dear Dr. Keith,**
>
> **I am a gay male. When I am indulging in my favourite activity (I am a topper), I always get an onset of leg cramps just before the rush to ejaculate. These cramps are sometimes very debilitating. Needless to say, they are counterproductive to the activity at hand, and the situation can have a negative effect on a relationship.**
>
> **I exercise four to five times a day. I don't smoke. I drink very little (one beer per week max), and I don't eat red meat of any kind. At first I suspected the leg cramps might be connected to my diet; however, now I don't believe this to be the case.**
>
> **Do you have any advice for me? My family doctor is at a loss.**
>
> **J.-C.**

Dear J.-C.,

Sounds like these cramps are a bit of a mystery, especially if they are occurring only before orgasm. I'm assuming your family doctor has done the basic blood tests and checked for electrolyte imbalances, which could be one cause. However, unusual problems like this are often caused by a combination of things.

What I wonder is if you are overdoing it with the exercise. Four to five times a day is a lot of exertion on your legs, and overworked muscles are prone to cramping. Any supplements or medications you might be taking to keep up this level of activity could also be to blame. You could try putting your legs in different positions before you come, to see if it's their position that's causing the cramping. If that doesn't work, try cutting back on your exercise routine to allow your legs some rest time, and see if this makes any difference.

If all else fails, you might consider a consultation with a specialist in an area like sports medicine or rheumatology, to see if he or she could give you some insight or perform any specialized tests that might be helpful.

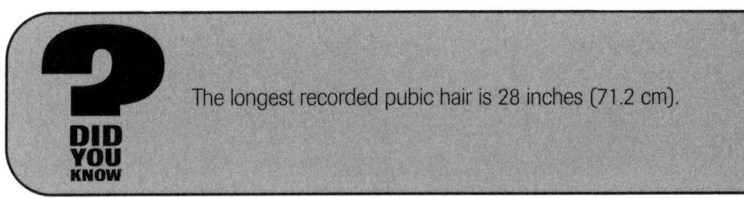
The longest recorded pubic hair is 28 inches (71.2 cm).

**❝ Dear Dr. Keith,**

**I'm not so sure I understand these butt plug things. Are they for when you've taken too many fists and you're worried about what might fall out? ❞**

**Tommy**

Dear Tommy,

The word "plug" in this case does not actually mean that a butt plug's purpose is to hold anything in, like the plug in a sink full of water. A butt plug is a sex toy similar to a dildo; it is often bulb-shaped, tapered into a smaller tip. It can be used for anal stimulation or to gently dilate the rectum in preparation for penetration and/or intercourse. You should always use one shaped in such a way that it can't be lost inside the rectum (a plug with a wide, flat base, for example)—who needs an embarrassing trip to the ER? It's also important not to use such devices if they cause pain or bleeding, warning signs that something is not right. If that happens, seek appropriate medical follow-up. Otherwise, enjoy.

> **Dear Dr. Keith,**
>
> **Can you please share with me some things I could do to bring the new man in my life pleasure? His member is a solid 8-plus inches (20-plus cm) uncut. I would love to swallow all of it. However, I am very new to gay sex and have only played in the minor leagues up to this point. Please help me to offer him the pleasure he is able to give during oral sex.**
>
> **Nino**

Dear Nino,

Welcome to the majors! Oral sex is an art form, and you usually get better at it with experience.

The most important thing you can do now is to be honest with your man. Explain that you are new to the blow-job scene. But emphasize how much you want to get him off with your mouth, and ask him to guide you. It can be very, very sexy if you both are into a little student/teacher play.

Hopefully he can guide you as to what he thinks feels good. But, as a general rule, start off by getting used to how the tip of his penis feels in your mouth (the head, or *glans*, is the most sensitive part), using your tongue, sucking, kissing, and making in-and-out motions. Gradually work your way back, taking in as much as you can. Gagging may be a problem, but there are ways to work around this (see the next question). Use your hands to complement the work you are doing with your mouth. And always, *always* watch out not to apply your teeth too heavily; use your lips to shield them while you suck him in and out of your mouth. Some use of teeth can be good, but this takes experience and direction from your guy.

Find out what others do by conducting a little research. There are some great books and on-line references out there. Plus, it's always a good idea to compare notes with friends. Everyone has a different style and different experiences.

Communication (as always) is the key here. If you want to please your partner, you need to find out what he likes. With some guidance you'll be able to deliver. You can never go wrong with that kind of approach.

Happy slurping!

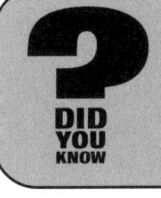

> In Charles Panati's book *Sexy Origins and Intimate Things*, his list of well-endowed twentieth-century celebrities includes Arnold Schwarzenegger, Jason Priestly, Charlie Chaplin, and Frank Sinatra.

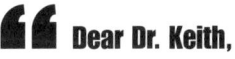

**Dear Dr. Keith,**

**I constantly gag when trying to suck cock. What can I do? It is totally cramping my style, and the last thing I want is to barf all over some hot guy's dick.**

**Martin**

Dear Martin,

That pesky gag reflex—it's a problem for many men. I agree; unless you're in a kinky situation that calls for it, vomiting on your man's penis is not cool.

We gag when the sides and back of the throat are touched. (This is why some people stick their fingers down their throats when they want to vomit.) Some people are more sensitive than others. So avoiding contact with these areas is one approach.

Try repositioning first. Many guys, with great success, have tried lying on their backs with their head hanging over the edge of the bed, so that the neck and head are tilted backwards. (This is a position similar to that used by sword swallowers!) Other positions may work, too; you'll have to experiment to find which ones are best for you. The important thing is to keep your partner's penis centred in your mouth to avoid touching the gag areas.

Lozenges and throat sprays containing anaesthetic, intended to treat sore throats, can also be useful. These work by numbing your throat, so that your gag reflex isn't activated. The downside is that you can't feel or taste anything, two of the perks of blowing someone. You might also numb his penis, making things even more difficult.

If all else fails, try doing other things besides deep-throating, concentrating on the part of the penis you can get into your mouth with no problem. This is the most sensitive part of the penis anyway, especially the head. Kissing, sucking, nibbling, blowing, licking: all of these actions can be used to turn your partner on. Ask him what he likes. Use your hands, too. Following your hands up and down when taking him in and out of your mouth usually feels very nice. You can invariably find some way to drive him crazy without having to swallow his whole erection.

Play around (literally!) and you will find your own best style…and have fun while you're doing it.

> **Dear Dr. Keith,**
>
> **I am a 21-year-old gay male, and I masturbate a lot. Most of the time I masturbate using my hands. Sometimes I use a different technique (putting my penis between mattresses to simulate fucking). My average is four to five times a day, although sometimes I get up into the double digits. Is this normal or do I just have a high sex drive?**
>
> **I also like to use a dildo to stimulate my prostate while I masturbate, which increases the pleasure tremendously. However, on a few occasions, I have experienced a sharp pain while doing this. Is this normal?**
>
> **Richard**

Dear Richard,

Masturbation is a natural, healthy practice and no occasion for shame. The majority of men, both straight and gay, masturbate periodically throughout an average week. While I was unable to find good scientific data, some sources estimate that the "average" man masturbates approximately eight times a week, with a higher incidence in adolescents, when testosterone levels skyrocket, and a lower incidence in older men, when testosterone levels are gradually decreasing. Of course, large variations can exist between one guy and the next. Like yourself, many men use prostatic stimulation to heighten the pleasure of masturbation.

The frequency you report of four to five times a day may be considered by some to be excessive. As long as it isn't causing problems with your day-to-day functioning or affecting your sexual relations with others, then it is probably a non-issue. However, if it is causing impairment of any kind, you might want to consider the possibility that you have a sexual addiction. It's worth discussing this with a physician or a counsellor.

As to your question about sharp pain during anal play, any pain you experience when penetrating yourself should be treated as a warning bell. Pain usually indicates that something is wrong, and you should stop what you are doing. Blood is another cause for alarm. If you are repeatedly experiencing rectal pain, you should be examined by a physician to determine that the cause is not infection, fissures, or some other treatable condition.

Hope this helps!

---

**DID YOU KNOW**
The average number of times a man will ejaculate in his lifetime is said to be 7,200.

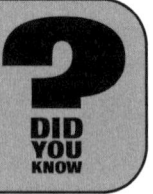

---

❝ **Dear Dr. Keith,**

**My name's Andrew. I'm 17 and I'm gay.**

**I'm a semi-closet case, and I live in a small town. It's really tough being gay here, so I have a lot of questions, opinions, and feelings that I keep to myself. However, I'd like to ask you a few things, some of which may sound stupid. You're a doctor, so I'm sure you're used to it.**

**Are cock rings dangerous? I've heard that, because they**

unnaturally restrict blood flow, they can cause damage to your penis. Is that true? And if it is, what kind of damage?

Finally, how do our bodies make cum, and what's its nutritional value? **"**

Andrew

Dear Andrew,

Great questions. The first one is easy: the answer is yes, cock rings can be dangerous if not used properly. You are absolutely correct: they act by strangulating the penis, keeping the blood inside the expandable tissues. This causes the penis to stay engorged and stiff. While this may be satisfying to some men because it maintains their erection, keep in mind that a cock ring also restricts new blood from entering the penis—imagine wrapping an elastic around your hand. Prolonged use of cock rings can cause damage to the nerves and blood vessels in your penis. They should therefore be used carefully, ensuring they are not too tight, and only for short periods at a time.

I had to research the second part of your question. What I found seems to indicate that the average male produces around 1 teaspoon or 3.5 mL of cum per ejaculation. That's the average, meaning 50 per cent of guys have more and 50 per cent have less. Ejaculate consists mostly of sperm (made in the testicles), seminal fluid (from the seminal vesicles), and prostatic fluid (from the prostate gland). According to a wide range of questionable sources, the average calorie count in one ejaculation ranges from 1 to 15 calories. One source even claims that one ejaculation provides 3 per cent of your recommended daily intake of zinc. I have no comment on how accurate that might be!

> **DID YOU KNOW**
>
> The longest medically recorded ejaculation travelled is 11.7 feet (3.4 m).
>
> The average speed of a male ejaculation is 28 miles (45 km) per hour.
>
> The average ejaculation contains 200 million to 600 million sperm. Anything less than 50 million can result in fertility problems.

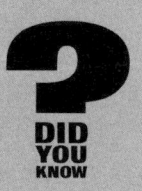

# A Queer Quiz

**1** According to this psychologist, we are all born bisexual and have an unconscious opposite gender hidden within us; the role of this archetype is to guide us towards the perfect mate.
  (a) Sigmund Freud
  (b) Carl Jung
  (c) Erik Erikson
  (d) Lawrence Kohlberg

**2** This team began research on sexuality in the late 1950s, and their work included watching men and women having sex and masturbating. They were also one of the first scientific collaborations to debunk homosexuality as an illness.
  (a) Smith and Klein
  (b) Laurel and Hardy
  (c) Masters and Johnson
  (d) Watson and Crick

**3** Gay or lesbian parents are more likely to have a queer child. True or False?

**4** Viagra works by:
  (a) Causing neurochemicals to be released in the brain, which creates sexual excitement
  (b) Dilating blood vessels in the penis
  (c) Causing the skin on the penis to be more sensitive to stimulation
  (d) An unknown mechanism

**5** Having an erection for too long is an emergency and is called:
- (a) Erectus longus
- (b) Steel-shaft syndrome
- (c) Euphoria
- (d) Priapism

**6** Which celebrity has talked about his third nipple in interviews?
- (a) Pierce Brosnan
- (b) Brad Pitt
- (c) Mark Wahlberg
- (d) Tom Cruise

**7** What is the medical word for involuntary vaginal spasm?
- (a) Vaginismus
- (b) Spastic vagina
- (c) Cloacal hypercontractility
- (d) Quiverism

**8** What frequently quoted gay nineteenth-century playwright died from a serious ear infection in 1900?
- (a) William Shakespeare
- (b) Michel Tremblay
- (c) Oscar Wilde
- (d) Christopher Marlowe

**9** The word "gay" was first used to describe homosexuality in Gertrude Stein's novel *Miss Fur and Mrs. Skeene* in 1922. True or False?

**10** What famous gay ballet dancer from Russia, who died in 1993, initially defected to France out of fear for his life?
   (a) Anton Kirov
   (b) Rudolf Nureyev
   (c) Mikhail Baryshnikov
   (d) Boris Yeltsin

**11** The word "lesbian" comes from:
   (a) The Isle of Lesbos, where a famous all-girls school was founded in ancient times
   (b) The Greek word *lesbon*, which means "strongly female"
   (c) The mythical goddess Lesbia, who protected the sovereignty of women
   (d) The acronym LSBN which stood for "lovely, smart, butch, non-male"

**12** In 2003, scientists found a gene that, when inherited, causes homosexuality. True or False?

**13** Which is more infectious, Hepatitis B or HIV?

# Answers

**1** (b), **2** (c), **3** False, **4** (b), **5** (d), **6** (c), **7** (a), **8** (c), **9** True, **10** (b), **11** (a), **12** False, **13** Hepatitis B

# 3
# Girl Parts

**Oral sex, dildos, clits, and more**

**THE CLITORIS** and the head of the penis have an equivalent number of nerve endings. But since the clitoris is smaller and more compact, it is much more sensitive to stimulation.

❝ **Dear Dr. Keith,**

**My girlfriend can't be penetrated by anything longer than 5 or 6 inches (13 to 15 cm). We want to use longer toys, but they hurt her. Is there some way of fixing that?** ❞

**Keli**

Dear Keli,

The depth of the vagina is not flexible. Unlike the vagina's diameter, which can be gently stretched over time to accommodate larger things, there really is no way to make the vagina significantly deeper. Vaginal length is determined by the distance from the vaginal opening (the introitus) down to the area beneath the cervix. On average, vaginal length is about 3 to 5 inches (8 to 12 cm).

Painful sex can be caused by an abnormality in the vagina or cervix. Pain on penetration can also be caused by an infection, an injury, or vaginal dryness. These things can most likely be treated, and they are important to rule out.

Assuming that the vagina is healthy, however, you must play with what you're dealt. So the best thing would be for you and your girlfriend to alter how you play. Deep penetration is not necessary for good sex. In fact, if you think of the vagina as being divided into thirds, most of the sensation rests in the third closest to the vaginal opening. So concentrate on that area instead.

❝ **Dear Dr. Keith,**

**I am a divorced 37-year-old woman, and I have just settled into my first relationship with another woman. We have had oral sex,**

**but I have never been able to make her come. She has to do it herself. Teach me!** 🙸

**Anna**

Dear Anna,

The best person to teach you is not me. And I'm not just saying that because I'm a gay man. The person who can help you most is your partner herself. It's her body; nobody has more experience with how to make her orgasm than she does. So ask her! Outside of the bedroom, strike up a light conversation about sexual experiences and share with each other the things that you really like. Then take that back to the bedroom. Tell her you want her to come, and that you want to help. Watch her masturbate a few times. Then, the next time, help her out. Let her guide you to what she likes and dislikes. She'll tell you, trust me. As long as you keep it fun and intimate, you really can't go wrong.

A few tips to get you started from what I've learned: first, it's all about the clitoris. For each woman, there exists a perfect balance for the stimulation of that important little friend; too much can be uncomfortable, too little leads to boredom. So pay attention to how much your partner likes and use your fingers, tongue, or objects to get her going.

Second, mood and state of mind are crucial. Make things sexy and fun; get her excited by teasing. Caress and kiss her thighs, neck, nipples, belly, and back. Anticipation makes sex all the hotter. And then, as my friend Ange says, "Go for the main course."

---

The longest recorded clitoris is 4½ inches (11.4 cm) long.

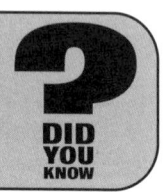

**DID YOU KNOW**

> **Dear Dr. Keith,**
>
> **Why is my clitoris so big? I find it embarrassing. Can I have it reduced like some girls do to their breasts?**

    **Emily**

Dear Emily,

The clitoris is like any other part of the body—there is a lot of variation. Like noses, feet, hands, and nipples, the clitoris comes in many different shapes and sizes. And like the head of the penis—I hope you won't mind if I make the comparison!—the "clit" engorges with blood during sexual excitement and increases in size. Some clitorises get bigger than others. Again, everyone is different.

    Can the size of your clitoris be changed? No. My advice is to relish what you have. A big clitoris is not only impressive to some women but a sign of enhanced prowess and even stature in some cultures.

    My question to you is this: if guys who like big penises are called size queens, what are girls called who like big clitorises? Size kings? Food for thought.


> **Dear Dr. Keith,**
>
> **I am in a long-standing relationship with a woman, and I have a question for you. When my partner has an orgasm, she ejaculates like a man. Is this normal? I don't ejaculate when I have an orgasm. I am just curious about this.**

    **Christie**

Dear Christie,

It's important to remember that while people are built similarly, we all work a bit differently. As with men, when women orgasm the difference in the amount of fluid produced can vary greatly, from none at all to copious amounts—all of which is normal.

It's interesting to note that female ejaculation is a subject of debate in the medical community—gynecologists and urologists can't seem to come up with a definitive answer as to its source. Men have glands, including the prostate, that produce most of their fluid on ejaculation, but women do not have these. Many experts will argue that female ejaculation involves the involuntary release of urine, but this is unsubstantiated.

No cause for alarm, however. Whatever the source, this release of fluid is natural. Many women out there are likely envious.

> **Dear Dr. Keith,**
>
> **What's a pussy fart?**
>
> **Shannon**

Dear Shannon,

A "pussy fart" is what we medically call "vaginal flatulence." Let me explain that in English. When air builds up inside the vagina through the repeated movements of vaginal penetration, the air pressure eventually becomes so high that air escapes back through the vagina. This causes the soft skin of the vagina to vibrate and create sound. It is very much like passing wind, or farting. It is normal, and to be expected. Girls, don't worry—it happens when guys are penetrated, too.

Happy farting!

> **Dear Dr. Keith,**
>
> **I often find myself dry when my girlfriend is using toys on me. It wasn't like that when I was younger. I am 52 now. Should I worry?**
>
> **Tanya**

Dear Tanya,

No, you shouldn't worry. As women age, especially during and after menopause, they lose a lot of vaginal lubrication. This is caused by decreased hormone levels in the body. Your dryness is likely part of this natural process. Ask your doctor during your regular check-up to do a quick exam to ensure there is nothing else going on. Then ask her or him about your options. Hormone Replacement Therapy (HRT) can be helpful for vaginal dryness, but at the current time it is controversial, since it might be more harmful for women than once thought. Local hormone creams might be an option, but good old-fashioned lubrication would be your best bet to try first. Some lubes can be irritating, so avoid those containing glycerine/glycerol and nonoxyl. Both compounds have frequently caused problems for women.

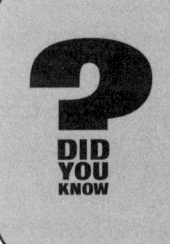

**DID YOU KNOW**

Beverly Whipple, a certified sex educator and counsellor, and John D. Perry, an ordained minister, psychologist, and sexologist, named the G-Spot after gynecologist Dr. Ernest Grafenberg. Dr. Grafenberg did not call it this when he first wrote about it in a 1950 article appearing in the *International Journal of Sexology*.

❝ Dear Dr. Keith,

I noticed my breasts are really tender during sex sometimes. During my periods, it seems worse. My doctor said not to worry, and she won't do a mammogram because I am only 22. I am terrified it's cancer, though. What do I do? ❞

    Winnie

Dear Winnie,

Increased breast tenderness just before and during your menstrual periods is common, due to the fluctuation in your hormone levels at that time. If the tenderness is in both your breasts and not in one isolated area, and there are no suspicious lumps, then the tenderness is no cause for alarm.

    As to your concerns about your family doctor's decision: unless you had a family history of breast cancer occurring at a young age, I would likely not do a mammogram either. Mammograms in younger women are often difficult to read, due to the highly dense tissue in their breasts, and accordingly they are not very useful. However, if you are still anxious about this and think that a mammogram might make you feel better, then you might ask your doctor about it again.

❝ Dear Dr. Keith,

My girlfriend says I get bitchy a lot, and she can't stand to be around me. She says that I must have PMS and that I need to take the Pill. Can you tell me more about it? ❞

    Kerri-Anne

Dear Kerri-Anne,

PMS has unfortunately become the target of jokes, but I assure you it's not funny for those who actually suffer from it. It's a monthly occurrence of various physical and emotional symptoms that are connected to your menstrual periods. The exact cause is unknown, but PMS is thought to be related to many things, including fluctuating progesterone levels and nutritional deficiencies. Women who suffer from it often complain of fatigue, irritability, depression, crying spells, pain, or bloating, although there are many, many more symptoms as well.

Treatment for PMS varies, and while there is no proven "cure," many alternative therapies can be beneficial. These may include counselling, a change in diet, or herbal remedies such as St. John's Wort and gingko. Some women also report success with prescription medications like oral contraceptives, antidepressants, and anti-inflammatories. There are potential problems with taking these drugs, though. You should make an appointment with your family doctor or gynecologist to have a physical exam and discuss this further.

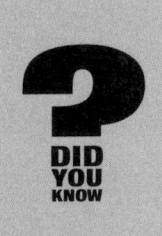

> **DID YOU KNOW**
>
> According to a medical book entitled *The Solitary Vice*, first published in the 1890s, women who masturbate are likely to eat foods with high concentrations of vinegar and mustard.
>
> According to *The Hite Report*, Shere Hite's groundbreaking study of female sexuality, the most common item women use for masturbation is a candle.

❝ **Dear Dr. Keith,**

Sometimes when my partner is sucking on my breast, I can have an orgasm without her touching me anywhere else. It's kind of cool, but is it some sort of weird abnormality? It doesn't happen to my partner. ❞

Laura

Dear Laura,

You'll be happy to know that you are completely normal. Oxytocin is a hormone secreted in your body in response to nipple stimulation, and has been referred to as "the love hormone" since it can by itself induce orgasm. For most women, however, it takes more than that to achieve orgasm, it also requires clitoral and vaginal stimulation as well. But rest assured, there is nothing wrong with you—as long as it's a positive experience, lie back and enjoy!

# 4

# Boy Parts

"What is this?" and "where did it go?"
to "measuring up" and "getting it up"

**THE LONGEST** medically recorded erection is 12 inches (30.5 cm).

> **Dear Dr. Keith,**
>
> I have a problem that's hard to talk about. My cock size is around 5 to 6 inches (12 to 15 cm). I would like to have a bigger cock so guys will like me more. Can you recommend anything to make my cock increase in size? I would like it thicker, too. I work out at the gym and my body is pretty nice, but my cock is too small. Can you help me?
>
> **Dennis**

Dear Dennis,

Why is that men are so obsessed with size? The size of your car, the size of your house, the size of your wallet, and, of course, the size of your manhood. Ah, manhood. The fact that the penis is often referred to by that term reflects how we as a society have equated it with masculinity and virility. The more penis you have, the more of a big, strong, masculine man you are as well. Right?

Wrong. I like to think that we have come a long way in realizing that there is much more to being male than the size of our sexual organs. And it looks like we might have. All the recent studies I've come across (formal and otherwise) show that the majority of gay men really don't care. Very few actually consider size when deciding if someone is attractive or not. Even if a guy did judge you on your size, would you really want to date someone that shallow? I think not.

Lastly, Dennis, your size is actually right on what is considered to be the average: 4 to 5 inches (10 to 12 cm) erect. That means half of men are smaller than this, half bigger. Again, not that it matters.

So don't go searching for creams and pills that don't work

or pumps that may injure you. Take pride in who you are as a person, and find someone who likes you for the rest of you.

> **Dear Dr. Keith,**
>
> **Could you please talk about the prostate in gay males over 40? What is the cause of an enlarged prostate? And do hot spices really affect the prostate?**
>
> Glen

Dear Glen,

The prostate is a gland in the male urinary tract that lies between the bladder and the urethra, the tube where urine exits the penis. The prostate is responsible for producing a significant portion of the fluid contained in ejaculation. Because of its position in front of the bladder and around the urethra, the prostate can slow or stop the flow of urination if it swells or gets larger.

The main cause of an enlarged prostate is simple aging. As we get older, our prostate gradually swells. The medical word for this is hypertrophy. Because it is a natural process, we call it "benign," thus the name attributed to it, Benign Prostatic Hypertrophy (BPH for short). With BPH, some men can experience difficulty peeing. Less frequently, the prostate can eventually block the bladder completely, requiring emergency intervention. Most men, however, have few or no symptoms, and their BPH is of no consequence.

A urinary tract infection can also cause enlargement of the prostate. Such cases often happen quickly, are very painful, and can be treated with antibiotics. A third and less frequent cause of enlarged prostate is cancer, which can grow inside the gland.

Whether or not spices affect the prostate is not an easy question to answer. Specific spices, like turmeric and curry, have been suggested as treatments for both BPH and prostate cancer. Other spices have antioxidant properties—basil, oregano, rosemary, and cumin, to name a few—although there is continued debate over the exact role antioxidants might play in the prevention of cancer. There are, however, no good medical studies supporting the use of nutritional supplements or spices in the prevention or treatment of prostate conditions.

On the other hand, spicy foods have been blamed for causing irritation to the prostate and the urinary tract. I don't know of any specific studies on this, but it makes medical sense that the compounds in spices that irritate your digestive tract could bother your urinary tract as they filter out of your body. If you are having recurrent prostate problems, you might consider monitoring your diet to identify offending agents, then eliminating them accordingly. It's worth a try.

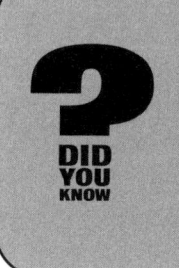

> **DID YOU KNOW**
> A eunuch is a man who has had his testicles (and perhaps also his penis) removed. It derives from the Latin word "eunuchus" which means "keeper of the bedchamber," because they were employed in ancient times as house-servants—hired to protect wives and children from romping around with the hired help.

**❝ Dear Dr. Keith,**

**I know a few things about the "A spot" for guys, but I was wondering if it is possible for a guy to ejaculate from the stimulation of his prostate if he's penetrated the right way. ❞**

**Terry**

Hi Terry,

The "A spot" is a part of the rectum that has gained infamy among males because of the pleasure that's often produced when this spot is stimulated during sexual activity. It was named after the G spot area of the vagina; stimulation of that spot is also reputed to be extremely pleasurable.

The A spot is located between your rectum and your penis, where your prostate sits. Massaging it gently can certainly produce enough positive stimulation to cause an orgasm. Prostatic massage leading to orgasm has even become a common running gag in Hollywood comedies.

## " Dear Dr. Keith,

### Is abstaining from sex bad for the prostate? "

Julius

Dear Julius,

According to a recent article in the *British Journal of Urology International*, men in their twenties who ejaculate more than five times a week decrease their risk of prostate cancer by a third. I must caution that other studies to date show only weak evidence of such a link, and in fact several of them have found there is no correlation. But if it's true, it would be great news for many guys.

And it's not just your prostate that may be helped when you are more sexually active. A 1997 study in the *British Medical Journal* indicated that men reporting a high frequency of orgasm had half the death rate from cancer of those who had orgasms infrequently. Other studies have suggested that having sex even a few times a week may lead to stronger immune systems, a better sense of smell, less heart disease, healthier teeth, less depression, less pain (including from headaches), increased fitness, and so on.

Meanwhile, there are those who assert that not "exercising" your prostate through ejaculation may make the gland more prone to infection. I don't necessarily think this is the case. And speaking of infections, remember that increased sexual activity increases your risk of sexually transmitted infections (STIs). So it is always important to protect yourself with condoms and safe-sex practices, especially since it's possible that gonorrhea and syphilis may increase your risk for prostate cancer. (The jury is still out on that.)

> **Dear Dr. Keith,**
>
> **I'm a 30-year-old gay man. I've noticed recently that my scent has changed. I find that I am not as "fresh" as I used to be. Why is that?**
>
> **Henry**

Dear Henry,

Interesting question. I'm not entirely sure what you mean by "scent," but I assume that you are referring to your skin, particularly around your genitals.

Your skin changes constantly over your lifetime. As you get older, it gradually thins. The production of oils changes, your hair thins and redistributes itself, etc. All of these things can change how the skin smells.

The skin around your genitals undergoes similar changes, and you will smell different over time. As long as it's not offensive, you shouldn't worry. If it is bothering you, washing down there regularly should take care of it.

" Dear Dr. Keith,

I am a 63-year-old man. Although I don't have a problem getting erections, I don't have much sexual feeling around my penis area, making it very hard to reach a climax. I started noticing this lack of feeling about ten to fifteen years ago, and it has grown worse. Now I have practically no feeling at all. I am having a real tough time because of this problem. I miss out a lot in my sexual life. I tried taking Viagra, but that only made me hornier and didn't give me any extra feeling. Could it be that I masturbated too much and wore off the end of the nerves around that area?

I have a few other medical problems, including my thyroid gland and high cholesterol. I take medication for both these conditions. I used to do shift work and had a hard time sleeping, so I started taking sleeping pills. I got addicted to those, and if I don't take them I just can't go to sleep.

What can be done about my problem? I would prefer not to talk to my doctor about this. I might be willing to go see a specialist, but what would a specialist in this field be called? A sexologist? I'm really anxious to start working on a treatment to restore those lovely feelings that make a person climax. "

Jason

Dear Jason,

I can understand the anxiety you must be feeling, and it comes across in the tone of your letter. What I hear you describing is a gradual decrease in your penile sensation over many years, which has often prevented you from reaching orgasm. This has nothing to do with you masturbating too much in the past.

Unfortunately, this is not an uncommon complaint. There are many causes of this decrease in sensation, including normal aging. It can also be seen in conditions like diabetes, malnutrition (vitamin B12 and folate deficiencies, for example), and neurological diseases like multiple sclerosis. Hypothyroidism, which you indicate you have, also can cause sensation disturbances. Other frequent culprits of sexual dysfunction are alcohol, recreational drugs, and prescription medications (blood pressure medicines, antidepressants, and anti-anxiety pills, to name a few).

In your case, the medication you take for sleep could be affecting your sexual function; this is often true of the Benzodiazepine class of drugs, frequently prescribed for acute sleeping problems and to calm anxiety (although impotence and loss of libido are the most common side effects). I would suggest getting off this medication with help from your doctor and exploring other options for your insomnia. Your doctor also needs to do a careful history and a physical that includes a neurological exam, along with some blood tests to assess if you have diabetes, if your thyroid medication levels are effective, and if you have other causes of neuropathy (nerve disease, which could cause loss of sensation) that can be controlled.

A urologist's assessment could be helpful and would likely include ruling out the medical issues I've raised above. Only a doctor treating you can make that referral, though, so you will need to consult a family doctor about your problem first.

It's worth doing the things I've mentioned to rule out reversible causes. However, I'm sad to report that all your efforts may be in vain, since the most common cause of the problem you're having is simple aging. I'm sure this is playing at least a part in your sensation complaints. If all else fails, experimenting with different ways of stimulating yourself to maximize your pleasure may be the only option available.

> **DID YOU KNOW**
> The average volume of male ejaculate over one lifetime is said to be 14 gallons (63 L).

> **❝ Dear Dr. Keith,**
>
> When I have sex, I have trouble reaching orgasm. It could have something to do with my age—I'm only 14. (Don't worry; I'm having safe sex with a guy close to my age who I really love and who really loves me.) It's just hard for me to reach orgasm when I'm having sex. Maybe you're thinking I'm not gay, but the prospect of a girl turns me off. When I get intimate with my boyfriend, I'm really happy. But it's annoying that I just can't reach peak. I hope you might provide possible reasons or things to help me. **❞**
>
> Rod

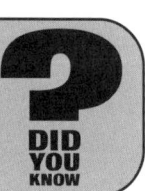

Dear Rod,

Inability to "peak" is often multifactorial, meaning there is usually more than one thing influencing your inability to reach orgasm. These reasons often fall into a few general categories, such as underlying physical disease; use of medications, including drugs and alcohol; and psychological issues.

For someone your age I'm guessing it falls into the latter category—psychological. No, I'm not implying that you are crazy, only that you are one of many people who can't seem to get into that right frame of mind. Sources of stress are all around us; some are obvious and some are not. Stress can affect how we function, including sexually. It affects our entire bodies, not just our minds; think about how your stomach tightens sometimes or how you start sweating in a tense situation. Stress throws our bodies out of balance, which can lead to inability to orgasm. When that happens we get frustrated, which results in more stress. Now you have more stress than when you started, which leads to more sexual problems, which leads to more stress, which leads to...

See where I'm going with this? Unfortunately, this is a common cycle that both men and women can lock themselves into. Somehow, the source of the problem needs to be identified and then dealt with. This often involves counselling with a trusted professional. Find a good therapist or doctor, and your problem should work itself out. In the meantime, explore ways that you can reach peak and then try to involve your partner. For example, if you find you are able to masturbate to climax with videos, do this a few times with your boyfriend watching. Gradually work your way up to touching each other, then eventually more. Take a step-by-step approach from what you *can* do and work your way slowly to what you *want* to do. And make it fun in the process!!

Good luck!

**❝❝ Dear Dr. Keith,**

**If a 51-year-old man has trouble keeping a full erection, is it because the levels of testosterone in the body have decreased,**

**or is it a mechanical problem with the little valves that are supposed to keep the blood from leaving the penis?** 💬
**Réal**

Dear Réal,

This is a very large question...excuse the pun!

Problems with maintaining an erection can have a psychological or physical source. Psychological causes can include loss of sexual arousal or interest, stress, mood disorders like depression, and fatigue. In these cases, your equipment is in working order and normal; it is just not getting activated properly. Given the right mental circumstances, everything returns to normal.

Physical or mechanical causes can include conditions in which the structures inside the penis are not working properly. The expanding tissues that make the penis erect may have been damaged through injury. The blood vessels that provide blood to these tissues may be damaged, perhaps due to diabetes or vascular disease caused by smoking. Or, as you stated, the valves that stop the blood from leaving an erect penis may be leaking, preventing the penis from remaining hard.

In some cases, something of a chemical nature may be interfering with the activation and maintenance of your erection. This is seen with hormonal imbalances such as testosterone deficiency (although that is uncommon) and thyroid disease. More frequently, the problem may stem from ingested substances like Ecstasy, alcohol, blood pressure medications, or antidepressants, to name a few.

Complicated, right? So how do you begin to decide what is happening? First make a trip to your doctor for a thorough history and physical, which should include an examination of the genitals, as well as the nervous system, and mood-disorder screening. In addition, you can distinguish psychological problems from physical ones by looking to see if you are still able to achieve a full erection during masturbation or have one when you wake up.

So talk to your doctor, and take it from there. He or she will likely suggest a trial of Sildenafil (aka Viagra) or a similar newer medication if it is felt you are a candidate.

Whatever the case, keep it up!

> **Dear Dr. Keith,**
>
> **Is Viagra safe for every male who has gone through puberty? Is there an age limit on its use? Also, what are the side effects of Viagra, and can Viagra make men without impotency have better orgasms?**
> **Clancy**

Dear Clancy,

Sildenafil, or Viagra, is a widely popular medication used primarily to enhance the ability to achieve or maintain erections. When a man is sexually aroused, the drug causes the blood vessels in the penis to dilate—get bigger—allowing more blood into the penis to make it hard. The drug works only when a man is turned on; taking the medication does not lead to automatic erection.

The side effects of Sildenafil most often reported are flushing of the skin, headaches, and stomach upset. Visual disturbances, such as sensitivity to light or even colour blindness (an inability to tell blue and green apart, for example), are also occasionally reported. More rare is "priapism," or sustained erection. This condition is very dangerous because it chokes the blood supply to the penis and can cause long-term damage. If it occurs, it warrants an immediate trip to the emergency department. Viagra should NEVER be used with poppers (amyl nitrate), nitrate-containing drugs, or substances like nitrous oxide or nitroglycerin, since the drug interaction can cause a potentially fatal drop in blood pressure. It's wise for anyone who takes other medications to discuss this with a physician, actually, to avoid other unwanted interactions as well.

Age becomes a factor if the person wanting to take Sildenafil has heart disease. While the direct effects of the drug on the heart are not well understood, sexual excitement can be very taxing for a weak heart. If you have heart disease, the medication should be used only under a physician's advisement. In fact, you should always obtain Viagra through a prescription from your primary doctor.

The jury is still out on the possible benefits of the drug for someone who has no problems with erections. There have been published reports of increased pleasure, particularly as experienced by women with a male partner, but the evidence is weak. However, the drug can act as a boost for someone who is lacking confidence, greatly improving his sexual enjoyment. In that situation, I believe in prescribing it, as long as the potential benefits outweigh the risks.

**❝ Dear Dr. Keith,**

**I have a testicle question for you. The first guy of the two I have been with only had one testicle. I found that very strange, but I didn't ask him about it, because I was shy and didn't want to hurt his feelings. Then I saw a guy with only one testicle in one of the Pridevision XXX movies.**

How common is this? Is the other testicle sometimes there but inside the body? The guy I was with was very sensitive around the area where his other ball would have been, and it really did take the fun out of it in a way. 🙌

Ken

Dear Ken,

There are a few reasons why one of a guy's testicles might not be inside his scrotum. The most common reason is that the testicle in question has retracted into the inguinal canal. This small passageway connects the abdomen and the scrotum, and it's the place through which the testes descend during a baby's development. Although the inguinal canal is not supposed to allow a testicle back into the stomach, sometimes the canal's outer ring is sufficiently lax to permit the testicle to "hide inside," making the scrotum appear empty. During periods of excitement, when the scrotum contracts (it is lined on the inside with muscle), the testicle can be pushed inside this space.

Another possibility is that the testicle hasn't descended while he was maturing in the womb. This condition is called "undescended testes," and it must be surgically corrected by bringing the testicle down. Otherwise, the risk of developing testicular cancer is increased. Occasionally, a testicle must be removed, either during childhood or during adulthood, for reasons including injury, torsion (spontaneous loss of its blood supply), or cancer.

If a man is physically sensitive to the touch there, be careful not to overstimulate the area. If having one testicle bothers him psychologically, and he doesn't want to talk about it outside the bedroom, then stimulate other erogenous areas of his body (his nipples, his penis, his armpits, etc.) instead. I had a patient with only one testicle who said his sexual partners sometimes even failed to notice that about him.

The main thing is to embrace each other's unique features, and enjoy!

> **DID YOU KNOW**
> Average erect penis size for a pig is 18 inches (46 cm). For men, it's significantly less: 4 to 5 inches (10 to 13 cm).

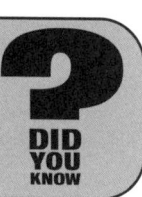

**❝ Dear Dr. Keith,**

**I have a recurring pain in one of my testicles. What could this be? My doctor gave me antibiotics for it once, thinking it was some sort of infection. The pain went away, but it still comes back occasionally. ❞**

**Hunter**

Dear Hunter,

Your doctor probably thought that a bacterial infection in your testicle or surrounding structures was causing the pain. Antibiotics are indicated in this situation. The fact that the pain resolved could have been from the treatment, but the pain could also have gone away on its own.

Your recurring pain warrants further follow-up from your family doctor or consultation with a urologist to rule out structural problems of the testicle and blood vessels, infections, and even cancer. A careful history and examination are needed, with appropriate investigations like urine testing and ultrasound imaging.

If these tests and the testicular exam are normal, then I would relax and chalk your pain up to the "phantom pain" many men experience, in which pain is mild, fleeting, and has no identifiable cause. Chances are this is your situation. But I wouldn't make that diagnosis until the other possibilities are excluded.

> **Dear Dr. Keith,**
>
> **Whenever I'm on the computer for long periods of time, the skin under my testicles starts to chafe. I think it's because of my leather chair. The skin gets very hot, itchy, and uncomfortable. Is there any way to prevent the chafing, or to cure it?**
>
> **William**

Dear William,

Chafing is how we describe skin breakdown and irritation caused by friction (rubbing). Doctors often see chafing of men's testicles due to underwear that allows the testicles and scrotum to rub against the leg. Thus the value of wearing properly fitted undergarments, which hug the scrotum close to the body and prevent friction.

Sweating can also increase the friction on your scrotum. Leather as a fabric does not "breathe" well—meaning air has difficulty passing through it, causing a build-up of moisture—so your chair is trapping sweat against your body. The combination of moisture and skin breakdown can even cause fungal infections around your groin, commonly referred to as "jock itch" by athletes.

You need to wear snug underwear and light clothing that

breathes. Spending less time in your leather chair would also help, as would covering the seat with a wool or cotton blanket. If the problem doesn't sort itself out, see your doctor and have him or her rule out a superficial fungal skin infection, which is easily treated with topical creams.

> **Dear Dr. Keith,**
>
> I have had a problem for years now. My testicles are very tender. I went to see my doctor about it, and he grabbed my testicles and pinched them. Man, was that sore! It was like someone had drop-kicked me right where it counts.
>
> The pain and uncomfortable feelings have been going on for some time, especially when it comes to sex. After doing an ultrasound, my doctor seemed to just write the whole thing off. I am worried about having cancer in my testicles. We have a family history of stomach and cervical cancer.
>
> What should I do?
>
> Paul

Dear Paul,

It's difficult to say what's really going on with your testicles, but I understand why you're concerned. When it comes to the "jewels," paranoia is easy to fall into. I speak for most guys when I say that nothing is likely to be more important to us than knowing our bits and pieces are in working order.

Testicular cancer is one of the most common cancers among younger men. It usually presents as a painless, growing mass on your testicle, and cancer can be detected with careful examination, blood work, an ultrasound, and a biopsy if necessary. To give you some reassurance, your doctor has examined you and done an ultrasound, and he was apparently not worried about the findings. If testicular cancer was causing your pain (and it usually does not), the cancer would likely be in only one of your testicles, and it probably would have been found by your doctor.

It's possible there's nothing physically wrong. You may just have developed increased sensitivity in your testicles over time, making them very delicate to touch. However, the possibility of a long-term, chronic infection needs to be ruled out. That can be done through simple blood and urine tests. You can also consult a urologist if no answers present themselves. The key thing here is that your complaint is not likely cancer, so relax, take a big breath, and try not to worry.

## " Dear Dr. Keith,

**Here's my problem: I am a senior, a retired teacher/school administrator. A few months ago, I noticed blood in my masturbate semen. It's been there ever since.**

**The sixty-ish husband of a friend of mine has the same thing. His urologist told him not to worry about it and said that it was the result of an over-supply of calcium. I've asked my doctor for a referral to a urologist, but I haven't been able to get an appointment yet.**

> I wonder if the calcium thing is legit. I've since cut out eating broccoli, something I was eating a lot of. **"**
>
> Ross

Dear Ross,

What you are describing is termed "hematospermia," or blood in the ejaculate. It is generally seen in men over the age of 40, although it can occur at any age, and it is usually due to a self-limiting inflammatory condition of the prostate or seminal vesicles (meaning it will go away by itself). While it can recur for weeks or months, the majority of cases result from a benign process and heal with no consequences. (Generally, more than ten episodes warrant further investigation.) It can be diagnosed after a physician conducts an appropriate medical history and a physical. If an abnormality is found on examination, or if the blood persists for months, this warrants an immediate referral to a urologist for consideration of diseases of the prostate, the bladder, or the rest of the urinary tract. Also (although rarely), in men over the age of 50, hematospermia can sometimes be a sign of prostate cancer. Since the blood in your ejaculate has persisted, I would recommend following up with the urologist as planned.

As for a possible calcium connection, after discussing this with a few urologists and doing my own research, I see no conclusive link between calcium consumption and prostate disease.

So, Ross... no cause for alarm, just make sure you follow up on it. And eat your broccoli, it's good for you.

> **"** Dear Dr. Keith,
>
> Help! My cum is frequently yellow and lumpy. That in itself isn't

**so bad, but my boyfriend tells me it tastes funny, too. Do I have an infection?** 🙣

**Carl**

Dear Carl,

Infections usually come on abruptly, and they usually cause pain on urination. Sometimes there is also a thick, yellow discharge present when you are not ejaculating. This discharge could indicate a sexually transmitted infection. However, if the fluid you're talking about is present only during sexual play, it has been there consistently for a long period of time, and it is not associated with any pain, then the chances are it is *not* an infection.

Normal ejaculate can change frequently in flavour, consistency ("lumpiness"), and colour. Your diet and fluid intake can greatly influence all of these things. Some foods, including vegetables, can not only cause pigment in your urine and ejaculate, but change the taste as well (asparagus, broccoli, and sugary foods have the latter effect, for example). Depending on how much fluid you drink and how often you ejaculate, the consistency of your ejaculate can become either more watery or lumpier.

A simple test from your doctor can rule out infection if there is any doubt.

# You like WHAT?

A condition in which a person's arousal and gratification depends on fantasizing about and/or engaging in sexual behaviour that is atypical is called a *paraphilia*. Match the following paraphilias with their source of arousal.

(1)  Plushophilia         (a) Feces
(2)  Hybristophilia       (b) Ghosts
(3)  Coprophilia          (c) Farting
(4)  Altocalciphilia      (d) Being a fugitive from the law
(5)  Klismaphilia         (e) Disabled elderly persons
(6)  Pedophilia           (f) Being in a large crowd
(7)  Emetophilia          (g) High heels
(8)  Gerontophilia        (h) Children
(9)  Hebephilia           (i) Enemas
(10) Ochlophilia          (j) Teenagers
(11) Spectrophilia        (k) Stuffed animals
(12) Eproctophilia        (l) Vomit
(13) Phygephilia          (m) Criminals

**Answers**
(1) k, (2) m, (3) a, (4) g, (5) i, (6) h, (7) l, (8) e, (9) j, (10) f, (11) b, (12) c, (13) d

# 5

# Sexy & Safe
## for the boys

**When your plumbing acts up**

IN 2003, 40 MILLION PEOPLE were estimated to be living with HIV/AIDS. Of these, 37 million were adults, and around 2.5 million were children under the age of 15.

**❝ Dear Dr. Keith,**

**Can you catch STDs from swimming pools or hot tubs? ❞**

**Lou**

Dear Lou,

No. By definition, sexually transmitted diseases, or STDs—the more common term now is STIs, or sexually transmitted infections—are spread by sexual contact. This means that the genitalia must come into close proximity with a potential source of infection, like the mouth, anus, vagina, or skin around the genitals. Also factor in that chlorine is toxic to both bacteria and viruses. You certainly can transmit an STI if you engage in oral or penetrative sex while in a pool or hot tub, but catching one because it is floating around in pool water is virtually impossible.

**❝ Dear Dr. Keith,**

**What is Staphylococcus aureus? And why is it so prevalent among gay men in North America? ❞**

**David**

Dear David,

Interesting question. Staphylococcus aureus, commonly referred to as "staph," is everywhere. It's on the ground, in your hair, on your skin, and up your nose (pleasant thought, right?). Like most bacteria, staph normally does not pose a problem unless it has a way into your body, such as a cut, a blemish, or an injury to the skin.

Staph got a lot of press at the beginning of 2003 when an outbreak of a particular strain was found in gay men in L.A., with growing numbers of HIV-positive men also being infected. A link to the bathhouses in the area was inferred. The key problem with this strain (thought to be related to a strain from France) was that it was highly resistant to the antibiotics commonly used in the treatment of staph infections. That made it exceedingly difficult to treat and caused considerable health problems for those affected. This specific strain also showed the ability to penetrate healthy skin, which is disturbing.

I'm not sure anyone is entirely clear why this S. aureus strain was particular to gay men. However, the outbreak provided an opportunity for the media once again to spin a negative story about the "saunas of sin" (that is an actual quote, believe it or not) where gay men spread bacteria to each other. Sigh.

The reality is that *any* antibiotic use will eventually lead to the development of drug-resistant bacteria in the future. Certainly that isn't a phenomenon restricted to staphylococcus. Many bacteria (including E. coli) are showing resistance to antibiotics today. So it's up to both the providers and the consumers of antibiotics to use them as sparingly as possible.

❝ **Dear Dr. Keith,**

**Is there a difference in safety between latex and non-latex condoms?** ❞

**Hiram**

Dear Hiram,

Latex can cause irritation and allergic reactions in some individuals. Non-latex condoms were created for these people. But all condoms in North America must undergo testing before being approved to go on the market, regardless of their composition. This means that although latex and non-latex condoms may feel different, and perhaps look different, too, the function of the condom is the same, and each is equally safe for preventing STI transmission (and pregnancy, for that matter).

> **Dear Dr. Keith,**
>
> **My boyfriend has been diagnosed with gonorrhea. We have been in a relationship for two years, and he tells me he has been monogamous. Is it possible to have got it from sitting on a toilet seat, as he claims?**
>
> **Jeff**

Dear Jeff,

Ah, the toilet-seat myth resurrected. The chances of catching gonorrhea from a toilet seat are so remote I'd say you're probably more likely to win the lottery three times in a row.

Gonorrhea is a bacterial infection transmitted to others by contact. It can infect your throat, rectum, or urethra, which means you can catch it through unprotected oral or anal sex. The symptoms range from a sore throat, anal soreness, and penile discharge to no symptoms at all. Gonorrhea is easily treated with antibiotics.

Someone has given your boyfriend the infection through a blow job or anal sex without a condom. One of two things has happened: he's been fooling around with someone else and caught it, or you have been the guilty party and spread it to him. (You need to see a doctor right away and get tested.)

Either way, it sounds as though your expectations for your relationship include monogamy, so clearly that's an issue here.

The two of you need to talk about the parameters of your relationship and about what kind of sexual activity with others (if any) is permissible. Remember, infections from oral sex can be prevented by using condoms, and that's not a difficult practice to adopt.

> **DID YOU KNOW**
>
> "Cold sores" and "genital herpes" are related. Herpes simplex virus-Type 1 (HSV-1) commonly causes cold sores or fever blisters on or around the mouth. Herpes simplex virus-Type 2 (HSV-2), which is only slightly different genetically from Type 1, usually causes recurrent lesions or blister-like sores on the genitals.

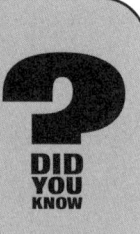

**❝ Dear Dr. Keith,**

**I have a huge problem, and I need some advice.**

**I've met this guy who is dying for me. At first we always had safe sex, with no penetration and no kissing. It seems so boring, but the fun part is that when we do Ecstasy we both enjoy our bodies, being touched, masturbating, playing out fantasies, etc. One day I decided to penetrate him bareback, but my penis only went in halfway, then I pulled out. Two days later I had this burning sensation on my prick and noted some whitish discharge. When I went to the clinic, they claimed that it was gonorrhea and not chlamydia. I was scared, especially when they said you are also likely to have HIV when you acquire gonorrhea, because of the capability of the bacteria to carry the virus with it.**

> I am presently taking doxycycline. Is this the right drug for gonorrhea? It's my third day of treatment and I still notice some whitish discharge, but it's dried out and stringlike at the tip of the penis. Is this normal? I have noticed that I have less pain and discomfort now.
>
> The guy I met claims that he is clean and also that he went to be checked and came out negative. Does this mean that I have had this disease in my penis for more than two days? Maybe months? If so, how come I didn't have any symptoms?
>
> Mike

Dear Mike,

Chlamydia is a bacterial infection similar to gonorrhea, in that both can be transmitted through oral, vaginal, and anal sex and both can cause discharge and burning. Doctors usually treat gonorrhea and chlamydia infections together, even if the test for only one of them is positive, since they often go hand in hand. You should have been given another antibiotic for the gonorrhea, since doxycycline is used for chlamydial infections. It will take a while for the discharge to disappear, so give it time.

As for how long you've had the infection, chances are you've had it for two weeks or less. Gonorrhea rarely takes longer than that to progress from the point of infection to the onset of discharge and burning. If your new partner is indeed negative (assuming they got a good sample from his rectum), then you have gotten the infection from other unprotected anal contact or a blow job.

Two final points. First, it is true that you are at higher risk for contracting HIV when you have gonorrhea or chlamydia.

That's because the infection irritates the lining of your penis, which may allow the HIV virus easier access to your bloodstream. However, you don't automatically have HIV just because you have one of these other infections.

Second, we should always be careful about maintaining safe sex practices when under the influence of alcohol and/or drugs, since these can impair our judgement and lead us to do things we normally wouldn't do.

> **Dear Dr. Keith,**
>
> I met a new guy recently. We have been dating for about a week now. All we have done so far is kissed, and he gave me a hand job and some head, but he disclosed a very serious problem to me, and I really need your help.
>
> This guy told me that he had gone to the doctor to get some anal warts removed last week. He went for his second treatment last night. Can you give me some information about them and how they're spread? Most of all, what are the dos and don'ts of fooling around with him? I don't want to put myself at risk. Apparently the warts were just anal, and his doctor told him last night that after one more treatment they will not be visible any more.
>
> Tell me what you think.
>
> **Ryan**

Dear Ryan,

Anal warts are caused by the Human Papilloma Virus (HPV). This particular virus can manifest in a variety of ways, from creating large finger-like warts to having no effect at all. The warts themselves can be many sizes, from too small to see to clusters of large, harder-to-miss ones. The virus is given to someone by touching, and it tends to prefer the genitals, the anus, and the perineum (the area between the anus and the scrotum or vulva). Often the virus is transmitted from person to person because the warts are not clearly visible. I've read recent studies that say, and even heard experts suggest, that the majority of sexually active men who have sex with other men are infected already, often unknowingly.

There are a few ways to treat warts. Toxic chemicals like podophyllin or trichloroacetic acid (TCA) can be applied by a doctor to kill them. They can also be frozen off with liquid nitrogen or burned off with a special tool. A medication named Aldara is sometimes used; it works by heightening your immune system, so that your body can rid itself of the warts. On rare occasions, warts are cut out using a scalpel or other such tool.

Some of these methods are more effective than others, as your doctor can explain. Regardless of these treatments, though, HPV has proven very difficult to cure, and it frequently comes back at some point. (Some specialists feel that you are never completely cured and so carry the infection in some form or another forever.) At a minimum, multiple treatments are required to get rid of warts appearing externally. Once the warts are no longer visible, the chance of infecting others is lessened, but theoretically infection may still occur.

One way to reduce *your* chance of being infected, Ryan (other than not having sex at all), is to use condoms. However, a condom will only protect the area that is covered, i.e., your penis. The more you have contact with this new guy, the more likely you are to get HPV. Presuming, of course, that you don't already have it.

However, don't let me scare you into abstinence—it's best not to let fear overcome you. Otherwise, we'd all stay at home with our doors locked. I'd suggest that you have no sexual contact with this guy until he finishes treatment, and then be careful to use condoms for any contact with his anal area, including penetration. Safe sex is always a good option. So: wait for him to finish treatments, then enjoy!

> **Dear Dr. Keith,**
>
> **I'm HIV positive and have been dating a herpes carrier. What steps should I take to protect myself?**
>
> Chad

Dear Chad,

The herpes virus, the culprit behind cold sores and genital herpes, affects a large percentage of the population. It causes irritating skin lesions that appear from time to time, then heal spontaneously. If you are infected, the virus lies dormant in your nervous system, resurfacing now and then to cause a "breakout." These breakouts occur for reasons not clearly understood, but they seem to be influenced by stress and illness, among other things. Sometimes people feel a breakout coming on by noticing discomfort or itching, which then proceeds to blister-type lesions. It's during these breakouts that a person is most infectious, so it's very important to avoid contact with your partner's lesions at these times. If you must have sexual contact, use barriers like condoms. However, using a barrier only works if the barrier covers the lesions, and it still carries some risk.

Once you have herpes, you have it for life. HIV can also

weaken your immune system enough that you could develop serious herpes infections should you contract the virus. In your case, I'd recommend abstaining from sexual contact from the time your partner feels an outbreak coming on until at least one week after the lesions heal. These would be great times to experiment with non-touching sexual situations like voyeurism. Might as well have some fun *and* stay safe, right?

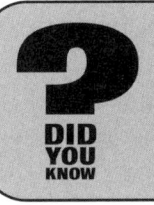

> **DID YOU KNOW**
> Circumcision removes the foreskin of the penis, and along with it an estimated 1,000 sensitive nerve endings. Many neurologists argue this makes circumcised men less sensitive to stimulation.

**❝ Dear Dr. Keith,**

**I have small red dots that I get all the time over the root of my cock and sometimes my balls. They never last long, but they always seem to come back. Is it herpes? ❞**

  **Pierre**

Dear Pierre,

It could be herpes. Genital herpes outbreaks present as small, blister-like lesions on and around your genitals. They disappear after a period of time, only to recur in the future. In order to diagnose herpes, these red dots would have to be examined by a physician and swabbed for laboratory diagnosis. The dots might not be herpes, though; they could be a condition called folliculitis, an inflammation of hair follicles that looks a lot like pimples. You could also be having a reaction to something that your skin doesn't like, like a lubricant or cream. Go see your doctor to be sure.

> **Dear Dr. Keith,**
>
> I was diagnosed as HIV positive last year. Although I've been able to talk about it with friends and family, and I have gotten a lot of support in this year, I'm still feeling a bit afraid when it comes to sex. Everything's changed for me. I no longer want to have one-night stands, and I'm afraid to tell guys my status when dating them, for fear of rejection.
>
> Some of my friends who are positive say that sex is between two consenting adults and you only have a responsibility to tell the other guy if he asks. Other friends advise taking it case by case. I've heard that most gay guys don't want to know and will assume that you're positive anyway. I'd like to believe that, but I know it's not exactly true.
>
> I still have a bit of anxiety when I don't tell my status, and now I'm sleeping with someone. What if the condom breaks? What if my sex partner has hep C or another STD and likes to rim? Do I tell or not tell?
>
> **Gerald**

Dear Gerald,

Whew. Great question, and one that could spark a series of ethical debates. You raise many interesting points and concerns.

Your fear of rejection is certainly understandable, because the chance of being rejected due to the declaration of your status is real. I wish I could say that the majority of men, if well educated, would not balk at the disclosure. Anecdotally speaking, however, my experience is that positive status is an issue for many men and might stop some from pursuing you.

That being said, my feeling is that any potential partner should know about your status before you have sexual contact with him. He has the right to know, since even though it's very uncommon to contract HIV through responsible sexual contact, the risk is still theoretically there. By disclosing your status, you give him a choice. By not telling him, you take away his right to choose.

This will likely lead to some men rejecting you. And that will hurt, guaranteed. But at least you won't feel you are deceiving the other person. And look at it this way—even if rejection does happen, wouldn't you rather share yourself sexually with someone who understands the situation, accepts the risk as small, and desires contact with you despite it all? That proves integrity, and perhaps dedication. Hopeless romantic that I am, I think those two things make sex much more incredible and meaningful. And you raise an excellent point about the mutual sharing of information: by avoiding disclosure to each other, you lose the opportunity to learn if he might have an infection that can be passed on to you. The last thing you need is another complicating infection.

My advice is to tell. It might close some doors for you, but you'll feel better about yourself, and you'll learn who's worth keeping around.

**" Dear Dr. Keith,**

**I have been in a relationship for over ten years. Two years ago I tested positive for HIV. My partner is negative. He still wants sex,**

> but I can no longer have sex with him because I'm afraid. I feel my life has taken a different turn, and I want to end the relationship. We have difficulty talking about most things. I want only to have a friendship with him. 〞

**Lucas**

Dear Lucas,

Becoming HIV positive can certainly be life-changing. I've watched many people take on a whole new attitude to dealing with living. Unfortunately, not all of these are good attitudes.

I'm sure that your partner being negative is putting a lot of pressure on you, and it is understandable that you fear giving him the virus. The fact that you feel so protective is wonderful. But—and I'm sure you've heard this before, but I'll try to reassure you again—having responsible, protected sexual activity carries with it a very minimal risk to your partner, and there is no reason to be afraid. He apparently doesn't have any hang-ups with your status, since he still asks for sex. And it sounds as if he has stood by your side since your diagnosis, which is a wonderful thing that sadly doesn't always happen.

So, are you wanting to break up with your partner because you're a changed new man or because you're afraid to infect him? If the latter is the reason, I'd advise you to seriously rethink your decision. A ten-year relationship with a guy as dedicated to you as your partner sounds doesn't happen every day.

If you just don't feel the same way about him for other reasons, though, then you probably do need to end the relationship. You say that conversation between the two of you is difficult, but in this situation it will be essential. Sit down with your partner to tell him how you feel and that you want his friendship. Hopefully, he will give it to you.

Either way, if you're still having difficulty handling this, there are many organizations out there that can help with counselling, some specifically for HIV-positive persons. Ask your doctor for a referral, or try searching on-line. The Resources & Acknowledgements section at the back of the book will give you a place to start.

> Dear Dr. Keith,
>
> I am hearing more and more about HPV and the importance of "pap" smears for gay men. Rectal cancer is a huge concern, since I have a family history of it. What are your thoughts/recommendations?
>
> Terry

Dear Terry,

You've hit on a topic that has recently become an interesting area of focus for physicians.

HPV, the Human Papilloma Virus, is acquired through direct surface-to-surface contact. While it's relatively harmless anywhere else on our bodies and in the environment, we know that if HPV infects a woman's cervix, it may cause changes in the lining there, and these changes could become cancerous.

Now, the same process is thought to occur in anal tissue exposed to HPV. Although scientists are still exploring the link between anal cancer and HPV, it is known that anal cancer rates are much higher in men with anal HPV infection. It is not known yet if women who practise anal sex might also be at risk.

A smear to detect anal changes is available to doctors for testing high-risk individuals, especially those with impaired immune systems (including HIV infection). This smear detects pre-cancerous cells in exactly the same way a female pap smear does, and corrective measures can be taken, if needed, to prevent the future development of anal cancer. Policies and recommendations are still being developed about who should be screened and when, but, at a minimum, HIV-positive patients should receive annual or bi-annual screening if possible.

Your original question asks about *rectal* cancer, though, which is a different issue altogether. If there's a history of rectal cancer in your family, I would strongly suggest having a discussion about this with your doctor.

> **Dear Dr. Keith,**
>
> **I'm 29 years old and married. Last weekend I had my first gay experience—I gave a guy a blow job. He's healthy and so am I. Could we get HIV? Does this mean I'm gay? Believe me, I get hard-ons just looking at a sexy man.**
>
> **Jack**

Dear Jack,

I'm hearing two questions here. You're wondering about HIV infection during oral sex. You also want to know if performing oral sex on a man means you're gay.

First, HIV is transmitted through bodily fluids like pre-cum, semen, and blood. In order for the virus to get into your body, it must have a way into your bloodstream. This usually occurs through small cuts or breaks in the skin. Although oral sex is considered to be less risky with respect to HIV infection, there is still some risk present. So your risk of getting HIV depends on whether or not your partner is infected with the virus,

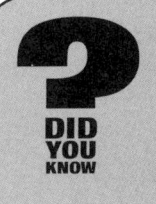

> **DID YOU KNOW?** Autoerotic asphyxiation, or cutting off the blood flow to your brain by strangulation, is said by some to enhance the pleasure of orgasm. According to U.S. government estimates, up to 2,000 Americans die every year from suffocation while trying this.

whether you were exposed to his pre-ejaculate or ejaculate, and whether or not there was a small break in the mucosa (lining) of your mouth at the time you gave him the blow job. If the answer to all three questions is yes, your chances then would be about one in a hundred, or 1 per cent. If you are particularly concerned, I would recommend HIV testing for you and your friend.

Second, are you gay? I don't know. Enjoying sexual activity with other men doesn't make you gay. What makes you gay is your *preference*. If you are turned on by other men, that's a pretty good indicator that you might be gay. Or you could be bisexual, if you have a genuine attraction to women as well.

Regardless, your confusion about your identity is both understandable and normal. What you need is people like you that you can talk to. Whether you find them on-line, at a bar, or at meetings is dictated by your comfort level. The broad world of homosexuality is a beautiful thing, so don't be afraid.

Good luck!

> **Dear Dr. Keith,**
>
> **Are bisexual guys and girls at lower risk for catching STIs than are gays and lesbians?**
>
> Gwyn

Dear Gwyn,

Your sexual orientation does not affect your risk of getting a sexually transmitted infection. Your sexual behaviour does. Your risk is determined by the number of partners you have had and the nature of your contact with them. For example, a gay man who always uses condoms and has had few sexual partners is at much lower risk than a bisexual guy who has had many male and female partners and occasionally forgets to use condoms.

So, no matter how you define or identify your sexual orientation, it's always important to practice safe sex.

# 6
# Sexy & Safe
## for the girls

**Why does it burn? Why do I itch?**

**FREUD FELT THAT THERE EXISTS** an unconscious belief in men that they may be castrated and lose their penis in the vagina during sex. He called this "vagina dentata," which translated means "vagina with teeth."

**❝ Dear Dr. Keith,**

**I find that there is little health promotion on STDs aimed at lesbians. So fill us in, will you? What is the truth about HIV? And what infections should we be concerned about? ❞**

**Samantha**

Dear Samantha,

You make an accurate observation. Education about STIs (sexually transmitted infections, formerly referred to as STDs), especially in the media, has tended to gear itself towards man-woman and man-man combos, neglecting the women who sleep with women.

Let's start with what we are *not* sure about. There is no well-documented case of HIV transmission from woman to woman through sexual contact. But that doesn't mean there aren't lesbians out there who have HIV; women who sleep with women are still contracting HIV through needle-sharing and sex with infected men. And there is some risk with sharing of toys. So the bottom line for women is this: DO NOT SHARE NEEDLES. And do not share toys without cleaning them or using condoms. And finally, if you're going to have sex with men, USE CONDOMS.

Now, let's move on to everything else. Hepatitis B can be transmitted sexually between women. Herpes can be transmitted through genital-to-genital or oral-to-genital contact. Trichomonas (which causes a foul odour, burning, and vaginal discharge) and the Human Papilloma Virus, HPV, which causes cervical cancer and warts, can be spread through penetration with fingers and toys. Syphilis, gonorrhea, and chlamydia are theoretically sexually transmissible between women, although this is rarely, if ever, seen. Lastly, any anal play (rimming or penetration) puts you at higher risk for Hepatitis A.

Protect yourself by using barriers during sex. Plastic food wrap works best, and it's nice because it can be torn to the size you want. Dental dams are a reasonable alternative, but they tend to be small, leaving uncovered areas exposed to possible infection. Hepatitis A and B vaccinations are easily obtainable through your family doctor or at a health clinic. (In some provinces these are provided free of charge. In others, unfortunately, they can cost a considerable amount of money, but it is absolutely worth the investment.) Cleaning your toys regularly and always using condoms on them is important if you share. Of course, not sharing toys is a sure way to prevent catching nasty stuff from "appliance use."

**❝ Dear Dr. Keith,**

**Is it possible to get genital herpes from your girlfriend going down on you if she has oral herpes? ❞**

**Sara**

Dear Sara,

Yes. Oral herpes, commonly known as "cold sores," is caused by a variant of the virus that causes genital herpes. There are many forms of the Human Herpes Virus (HSV for short). HSV-1 is found mostly on the face and/or mouth, while HSV-2 is a virus typically seen on the genitals or anus. But both viruses have the same predilection for sensitive tissues, so both can be transmitted to either place.

The worst part about herpes is that once you have it, you have it for life. It may not always be visible, but it hides in your nervous system and reappears periodically as blister-like lesions. Caution should therefore be used if you're having an outbreak, or if you feel one coming on. Abstinence and barriers such as condoms or dental dams are the best ways of preventing the transmission of herpes. There are medications available that you can take to suppress and treat outbreaks, and these may help reduce the risk of infecting others as well. Discuss these with your doctor for more details.

> **Dear Dr. Keith,**
>
> **I am confused! I am a lesbian, and I have heard conflicting things from my gynecologist and my family doctor. One tells me I have to have yearly pap smears, and the other tells me I don't need any. Who's telling the truth?**
>
> **Amy**

Dear Amy,

Until recently, both your doctors were right. More confused now? Let me explain.

Cervical cancer is strongly linked to a virus called the Human Papilloma Virus (HPV). This virus is sexually transmitted, and up until the last few years, it was thought to be transmitted through male-female sexual interaction only. Therefore, pap screening to catch HPV infection was not recommended for women who had never had male sexual partners.

New data, however, shows that HPV transmission does indeed occur between women, including those who have never touched a man sexually. So, therefore, a big YES to your question—you should get regular pap smears.

How often you are screened is up to you and your doctor, but I recommend getting the test at least every two years.

Perhaps it can be less if you're in a monogamous relationship and have had a series of negative smears in the past, but talk to your doctor. If she or he doesn't agree with performing a pap at all, find another doctor who will.

Cervical cancer is one of the only cancers that's truly preventable, so it's a tragedy in any woman, straight or queer.

> **DID YOU KNOW**
> The penis is relatively sterile (with the exception of organisms normally found on the skin). The vagina, on the other hand, is colonized by lactobacilli and often enterococcal and coliform species.

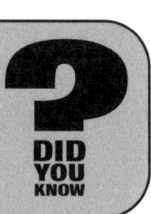

**❝ Dear Dr. Keith,**

**What is NGU? I was told by my doctor that I had it, but I am not sure what it means. Is it caused by sex or something else? I don't sleep with that many girls, and I don't have any other health problems. ❞**

**Stephanie**

Dear Stephanie,

NGU stands for non-gonococcal urethritis. This condition occurs when your urethra (the tube through which urine passes) becomes irritated and inflamed, for reasons other than a gonorrheal infection. NGU is most commonly caused by chlamydia, trichomonas, mycoplasma, and ureaplasma, which are all organisms transmitted through oral, anal, and vaginal sex, including the use of sex toys.

When your urethra is inflamed, it can cause burning, discharge, and painful sex, but NGU can also be asymptomatic.

Antibiotics are very effective for the most part in treating it. You can lessen your chances of catching it again by using a barrier like a dental dam or female condom for all oral and fingering contact. It is equally important to clean your toys before using them on someone else, or to use a condom on them, since sharing also spreads the infection.

> **Dear Dr. Keith,**
>
> **I find that I am most horny around the time of my period. I also find sex helps to ease my cramps. My previous partner had no issues about us having sex at that time, but my current partner thinks it is dangerous, and she is very nervous about being intimate then. What should I tell her?**
>
> **Sylvia**

Dear Sylvia,

Raging hormones around the time of your period are what make you horny, and that's fairly common. But the obvious concern here is the bleeding. Medical evidence concerning women who have sex with women and STIs is very limited. HIV and Hepatitis B and C can all be transmitted through contact with blood. While many consider woman-to-woman activity low-risk, there have been reported cases of these infections being sexually transmitted between women, and menstrual blood might have been a factor.

You and your partner should play carefully. If you're going to be active during either of your periods, then you need to prevent contact with menstrual blood as much as you can. This means avoiding toy sharing, unprotected cunnilingus (oral-vaginal sex), and unprotected penetration with fingers or tongue. Gloves, condoms on toys (do not reuse!), and dental dams are your best friends during your period.

With these precautions, the risk is minimal. If your partner is still uncomfortable with it, though, don't force the issue. Try no-contact things like watching each other masturbate, and over time she may change her mind.

## " Dear Dr. Keith,

I do a breast exam every month, and I have recently found that a bit of whitish liquid comes out of either breast. I have done some reading on the Internet and discovered that this can happen because of nipple stimulation. My partner often plays with and sucks on my breasts during sex. Is that a problem? Should I tell her to stop doing this? "

Angelina

Dear Angelina,

It's normal for some milk to be produced on nipple stimulation. As long as this isn't bothersome, it's likely to be fine, but it may still be a good idea to mention this to your health care provider to check that there isn't something else going on.

Also, be warned that breast milk does contain the HIV virus in infected persons. So you and your partner need to treat it as you would any other sexual fluid—with caution, until you determine that you don't have HIV. If you do, then you could possibly infect her through these secretions, so a barrier like a dental dam should be used.

❝ **Dear Dr. Keith,**

**Over the past year I have been getting frequent urinary tract infections. I had never had any before I became sexually active. They often occur after my partner and I have had sex, although not every time. Is the infection sexually transmitted? We try to be safe and use protection. How can I prevent this from happening?** ❞

**Leslie**

Dear Leslie,

Sex can cause urinary tract infections, or UTIs, by introducing bacteria into the opening of the urethra. Thus the name adopted by some to describe it: "honeymoon cystitis." Cystitis means inflammation of the bladder. Sounds romantic, eh? Not really! You can reduce your risk of getting a UTI by adopting a "clean routine," as follows: Use clean toys. Never allow a toy or finger in your vagina after it's been in your anus. Urinate before and after penetration. When wiping after a bowel movement, wipe front to back. Use lubrication to avoid dryness during sex. And avoid aggressive penetration. Doing these things will help decrease your exposure to the bacteria that can enter your urinary tract and cause nasty infections.

If this routine doesn't help, and you continue to get infections, ask your doctor to make you an appointment to see a specialist who can help rule out other things besides sex that might be at fault.

> **❝ Dear Dr. Keith,**
>
> I recently got my tongue pierced. I have been following the aftercare instructions given to me at the tattoo parlour where I got it done, but is there anything special or different I should do when I go down on a woman? Am I more at risk of getting something because of my piercing? ❞
>
> Jan

Dear Jan,

That's an interesting and thought-provoking question.

There's a possibility of getting a non-sexual infection in your tongue from the piercing, of course. The mouth is full of bacteria at the best of times. Keep your mouth as clean as possible, and avoid injuring the site further by pulling on it or playing with it. Because of the nature of the tongue, the wound around the piercing will take a significant amount of time to heal (some say weeks, others months).

Talking about STIs is different. A new piercing is an easy portal into your body for any infection it comes into contact with. That includes Hepatitis B, Hepatitis C, and HIV. Your risk if exposed to secretions or blood containing those is theoretically increased.

Although your risk is low (unless your partner is menstruating), you should avoid unprotected oral sex until your tongue is fully healed. Using a barrier may not be a lot of fun, but it will significantly reduce any chance of sexually transmitted infection. It never hurts to rinse with mouthwash after oral sex as well, although doing so beforehand can theoretically irritate the lining of your mouth and increase your risk.

> **Dear Dr. Keith,**
>
> I have an ex-girlfriend who called me and told me she had "trich." We had sex a lot, including sharing toys. What is trich, and what kind of problems does it cause? I feel fine.
>
> Dee

Dear Dee,

Trichomonas, or "trich" as it is commonly called, is a microorganism that loves the environment of the vagina and its surrounding structures. In some women the infection can be so mild that you have no symptoms; in others, there can be burning, foul discharge, and pain on penetration.

Trich is a common infection, and it's easily treated with antibiotics. Since it's passed around by contact with secretions, it's possible you've been infected from sharing toys or other exposure to your ex-girlfriend's vaginal fluid. Go to a clinic and get this checked out before you have problems or pass the infection on to someone else.

> **Dear Dr. Keith,**
>
> I am a lesbian, and my doctor told me to get a Hepatitis A vaccine, but I thought they were for gay men. Should I get vaccinated?
>
> Jenny

Dear Jenny,

Yes. Hepatitis A doesn't discriminate by orientation or gender. To be blunt, it is spread by contact with feces. Your body absorbs the virus through your digestive tract via your mouth or stomach, and it then goes on to infect your liver. As it replicates, it also infects your stool, and you can then pass it on to others.

Gay men are considered at higher risk of infection because they tend to be involved in anal play sexually. But being a homosexual man doesn't increase your risk; rimming (stimulating the anus with your mouth) and anal sex do. So *anyone* who does these things is at risk. Even if they don't "play in the back yard," lesbians should get vaccinated if they engage in oral-vaginal sex ("eating pussy") with other women. Because the anus is so close to the vagina, the potential exists to be exposed.

The vaccination is a simple series of two shots (three, if you're getting the combined Hepatitis A and B vaccine). It protects you while travelling, too, since contaminated water in less developed countries can give you Hep A.

> **DID YOU KNOW**
> The spotted hyena has such a large clitoris that in ancient times people mistook the clitoris for a penis. They thought the animal was changing from male to female and back again.

**❝ Dear Dr. Keith,**

**I get a lot of vaginal discharge in the mornings and always have. My new girlfriend is upset about it. She says it's chlamydia, and now she won't sleep with me. My doctor did swabs and she said it's not an infection, but my girlfriend doesn't believe me. What do I do? ❞**

Patricia

Dear Patricia,

Let's talk about the discharge first. Your girlfriend is right that chlamydia can cause discharge. Since your discharge has been happening for such a long time, though, and the swabs your doctor did were negative, it's not very likely to be chlamydia in this case. Normal vaginal lubrication, what we call "physiologic discharge," can often leak out in the morning, after a woman has been lying down all night. I'm assuming your doctor would have advised you if the swab had shown another STI, a yeast infection, or BV (bacterial vaginosis, a non-STI infection), all of which can also cause a discharge. So what you have is probably just normal secretions.

Your girlfriend sounds like she might have some trust issues. You and she need to discuss why she feels that your doctor is wrong. To reassure her, maybe you could ask her to accompany you to your next doctor's appointment (assuming your MD is queer-positive). If she's still not convinced, ask her what's really going on. Try to help her with whatever is bothering her, and work through it together.

**" Dear Dr. Keith,**

**How can I properly clean my sex toys to prevent me from getting infections? I used to use condoms, but they kept giving me yeast infections. "**
**Margaret**

Dear Margaret,

If you share toys during sex, condoms are a good solution to prevent the possible spread of infection. In your case, it sounds like the condoms you're using are irritating your vagina, causing inflammation. We call this "chemical vaginitis." The offending agent could be the latex or the lubrication and/or spermicide that is present in the condom. You might want to try latex-free, non-lubricated condoms and see if that helps.

The other solution—other than not sharing—is to use anti-bacterial soaps or bleach diluted in water to rinse your toys between users. This is cumbersome, however, and often not convenient during sex.

**❝ Dear Dr. Keith,**

**What are crabs? My ex-girlfriend called me and, out of hate, told me that she hopes she gave them to me. Could I have them and not know? And how do I treat them if I do have them? ❞**

**Amy**

Dear Amy,

Wow—sounds like there's a lot of tension and angry feelings between the two of you. Let's not address that now, since I have no way of knowing exactly what is going on.

What we do need to talk about is the crabs. If your ex-girlfriend had them when she was sleeping with you, you need to make sure you don't have them. Unfortunately, there's a 95 per cent possibility of contracting them after sleeping with an infected person even *once*. Crabs are related to body and head lice, but they mostly live in pubic hair. They live by feeding on your blood. After eating, they turn from a grey colour to a brownish-red and look like tiny crabs; hence the name. When you hear people talking about "nits," that's the eggs the crabs lay; they appear as tiny white dots at the bottom of individual hairs. On average, an egg will take between seven and ten days to hatch, although in unusual cases hatching can occur three weeks after the egg is laid. The crab can then live up to thirty days, laying more eggs and repeating the cycle. If crabs leave the body (going onto clothes, bedding, or towels), they will starve and die within forty-eight hours.

If you have crabs, you would probably know. The first sign is moderate to intense local itching. Check your pubic area for bluish marks where they may have bitten, for the crabs themselves, or for white nits at the base of your pubic hairs. Crabs can be present in your armpit hair, eyelashes, and head hair as well. (Men should also check chest hair and beards.) If you're still not sure, go to a medical provider and get yourself checked out.

Treatment for crabs is an over-the-counter body cream bought at the drugstore and applied for eight hours after bathing. (The treatment should not be used if you might be pregnant or are breast-feeding.) *All* of your clothing, bedding, and towels should be washed in hot water and put in the dryer if possible. If it's not possible to wash them, you can seal blankets and larger items in bags or even place them in your freezer. (The little guys hate the cold and die quite quickly.) You can expect itchiness and spots to last up to two weeks after treatment. Repeat the body cream only if you still find nits, crabs, or fresh bites after treating the first time.

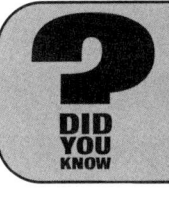

> **DID YOU KNOW**
> Some women are capable of "status orgasmus," a continuous orgasm that may last as long as 20 to 60 seconds.

**❝ Dear Dr. Keith,**

**I am constantly getting what my doctor calls BV. It is treated with antibiotic gel that's inserted into my vagina. I have heard that you can use yogurt as a treatment instead. Is that true? I would like that much better; I hate taking antibiotics. ❞**

**Kailey**

Dear Kailey,

Bacterial vaginosis, or BV, is caused by a disruption of the natural environment inside the vagina. That environment depends on a careful balance of the small amounts of bacteria that live there normally. When that balance is thrown out of whack, and certain bacteria begin to grow out of control, you get BV. The infection can cause a foul odour, vaginal discharge, and tenderness and itching of the vagina and vulva, although many women have no symptoms. The imbalance can be caused by antibiotics, douches, tampons, lubricants, diaphragms, or even semen, for women who have sex with men. (Semen disrupts the pH of the vagina.)

Antibiotics to treat BV can be taken as pills or applied locally in a suppository, gel, or cream. They are necessary as a first-line treatment if a woman is pregnant or planning to have a gynecological procedure done (for example, an abortion, a biopsy, or an endometrial ablation). Otherwise, it is reasonable to try a more natural remedy, such as inserting capsules of lactobacillus, the natural bacteria in yogurt, in your vagina at bedtime for one week. You can find these capsules at your drugstore or health food store. I wouldn't recommend yogurt itself, since it is so messy. Plus, some yogurts contain sugar and other ingredients that can cause more problems than you started with.

If the capsules don't help, try douching with a solution of one tablespoon of white vinegar in one quart of water before inserting the capsules. This will create a more acidic environment in your vagina, which may aid in restoring the natural flora. If the capsules and douching fail, go see your doctor.

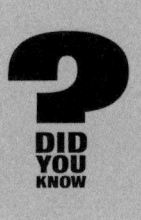

> **DID YOU KNOW**
> The inverted pink triangle, which has become synonymous with the gay community, was initially a symbol used by the Nazis to single out homosexual men for special abuse. Homosexual women were given black triangles, a symbol identifying them as criminals.

# What's bugging you?

Match the organism to the infection that it is caused by or associated with:

(1) Phthirus pubis
(2) Human papilloma virus
(3) Treponema pallidum
(4) HSV-2
(5) E. histolytica
(6) C. trachomatis
(7) Candida albicans
(8) Gonococcus
(9) H. ducreyi

(a) Chancroid
(b) Gonorrhea
(c) Chlamydia
(d) Yeast infection
(e) Genital warts
(f) Crabs
(g) Syphilis
(h) Genital herpes
(i) Amoebiasis

**Answers**
(1) f, (2) e, (3) g, (4) h, (5) i, (6) c, (7) d, (8) b, (9) a.

# 7

# What's Love Got to Do with It?

Questions about relationships

**LIKE MANY GREEK MEN OF THE TIME,** Alexander the Great (born in 356 BC) had many male lovers, and he is said to have staged one of the most lavish funerals in history when his male partner Hephaestion was killed in battle.

" Dear Dr. Keith,

I am 18 years old, and I have a question about relationship issues. I saw this guy at the gym one day and I knew there was something special about him. I kept seeing him there, and one day he came up to me and we started talking. I finally got the guts to ask him to go out for coffee. He agreed, and he also did something else, if you know what I mean. But we never really talked about it.

He was the first guy I have ever kissed, and I started to really fall for him. He had to go on a trip for work, so I didn't see him for a couple of weeks, but he phoned me from his hotel. So it seemed like everything was going well, and I assumed it was only a matter of time before we would start dating officially. But then things seemed to turn bad. He hardly ever phones me. He never wants to chill with me, because he's so tired from work, and I only get to see him at the gym. I don't know what to do. I don't want to hold the fact that he works against him; I'm happy he has a career and is striving for something in life. But he seems to be really busy all the time. I'm so scared. I really like him, but I don't want to seem too pushy.

I have never felt this way about anyone before, especially about a man. I would like to know if it's okay that I feel this way about him. Also, how do you know if a guy likes you back? I'm new to all of this and I just want to be understood and loved. 🗨

Jon

Dear Jon,

I feel for you, I truly do. Almost everyone has been in the same situation, myself included. You meet someone you really fancy, and he responds with similar interest. Everything seems perfect. Then, in the blink of an eye, something changes. The guy starts giving excuses for not seeing you; he keeps telephone conversations short; he stops holding your hand or wrapping his arm around you like he used to.

All this leaves you confused. You don't understand what's happened. You don't know whether he's reacting to something inside your relationship or whether his change of behaviour is due to something at work or at home (or maybe even in a relationship with someone else).

Regardless, the key to unlocking the anxiety in this situation is to remove the uncertainty. Talk to this guy about it and find out what has changed. Tell him that you've noticed a big difference in the way things are, and that you would appreciate his honesty. It's honesty you want, too; the last thing you need is him giving you some fabricated story in order to avoid conflict. With an honest answer on the table, you can decide if the relationship is salvageable.

If he isn't honest with you or doesn't want to talk about it, MOVE ON. That's easier said than done, I know, but things won't go back to the way they were. If the relationship is going to end, you need to accept that and get closure on it as quickly as possible.

It's not hard to tell that you really like this guy, Jon. If it works out, great. If not, what I can tell you is that the ache will go away; it won't always feel like this. There will be others who make you feel just as good, so, if necessary, let go of this guy and get yourself back out there. Find the next guy who makes you smile, the one you just can't stop thinking about.

> **Dear Dr. Keith,**
>
> **Here is my question for you: why do gay relationships seem so much more difficult than straight relationships? I am a 25-year-old-male looking for love, but almost all the men I meet are commitment-phobic, abusive, or addicted to drugs. I'm beginning to think about settling down with a woman. Please help.**
>
> **Colin**

Dear Colin,

Unfortunately, you will find people who are commitment-phobic, abusive, and reliant on drugs everywhere in society, not just in the gay community. There is certainly a stereotype that gay men are afraid of relationships, nasty to others, and interested mostly in snorting something or other up their noses. But this definitely isn't the norm.

There is a gay community that exists well outside of the clubs where these behaviours can predominate. And while clubs can be a great place for some people to meet potential partners, it can also be frustrating for someone like yourself. There are many other avenues available for meeting guys who conform to your preferences. Networking through friends, joining community activities, and placing ads on the Internet are all great ways of meeting people with similar interests.

I would also caution you against "looking for love." You'll

find it much less stressful if you concentrate on meeting people you're attracted to, and seeing where that takes you, instead of focussing on the end product. That kind of single focus can often lead to disappointment, making you less confident and even more frustrated than when you started.

Good luck!

> **DID YOU KNOW**
> When the human penis is stimulated, sensory nerve impulses travel to the brain at roughly 165–195 feet (50–60 m) per second. Similar nerve impulses in a cat reach speeds of 330–395 feet (100–120 m) per second. (I'll refrain from making a pussy joke here.)

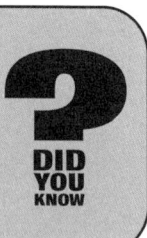

**" Dear Dr. Keith,**

**How do you know it's time to move in with your girlfriend? "**

**Marcia**

Dear Marcia,

Let me start off by saying this: you'll know when it's time.

One of the biggest mistakes a couple can make is moving in together too soon. Make sure that you and your girlfriend want to cohabit for the right reason—that both of you want to share a living space and spend more time together. Don't make the move because it's convenient or because someone is pushing you to do it. Decisions made for those reasons carry with them certain failure.

Talking about every aspect of cohabitation in advance is critical. Work out what the costs will be, and who is paying for what. Decide where you are going to live and who is going to provide which furnishings. Talk about responsibilities like cleaning, walking pets, grocery shopping, and cooking. Leave no stone unturned. I would also recommend a trial period of living together before committing yourselves. Live in her place for a while, or vice versa. This will give you a chance to learn more about each other and to discover each other's inevitable annoying habits. Developing and maintaining good communication through this trial period, along with understanding and empathy, can only make your relationship stronger and more successful.

Remember too that many successful couples don't live together. Being a couple doesn't necessarily mean that you have to. Some people are better off maintaining their independence, particularly with regard to living spaces.

In summary: think, talk, plan, and try. If it's right, go for it!

> **Dear Dr. Keith,**
>
> **I am a 20-year-old guy and am dating this girl who is fantastic. I am really into her emotionally, and our relationship is very strong. I have always fooled around with guys in the past, though. I want to play "the other side" but don't want to betray my girlfriend. Would you consider this to be cheating?**
>
> **Ramon**

Dear Ramon,

I think the question you need to ask yourself is, "Would my *girlfriend* consider this to be cheating?" The answer might be yes, and in that case you should avoid indulging your "other side." However, the only way to be clear on what her boundaries are is to ask her. You never know—she might not mind you sleeping with guys, as long as you are honest. If she's open to it, you could encourage threesomes with her and another man as a way for you to scratch your itch. But it's very important to clarify things with her before trouble erupts.

> **Dear Dr. Keith,**
>
> **I want to know why my partner feels he needs to sleep around. I am happy to have one guy, but he is not and I have a problem with this.**
>
> **Guy**

Dear Guy,

You are describing a situation that frequently causes conflict for gay couples. It's normal to have the desire to sleep with others. Some men indulge these desires secretly, while some do it with their partner's knowledge. Others prefer to repress the urge and stay faithful.

I know many male couples who have "arrangements"; both partners are allowed to have sex with other men as long as they respect the rules agreed upon by the two individuals. This approach works for some. But not everyone can, or wants to, run their relationship this way. Clearly, it's not an idea that appeals to you.

My advice to you is this: tell your partner you are looking for an exclusive situation. If he agrees, fantastic, although be careful that he is not just telling you what you want to hear. If he says he wants to sleep around despite how you feel, get out of the relationship. That sounds harsh, I know, but you'll save yourself a lot of heartache in the end. It sounds as if you are unhappy already, so maybe the time is right to rejoin the singles scene and find another guy with a predisposition towards monogamy.

> **Dear Dr. Keith,**
>
> **In the gay community, many men (if not most) seem to confuse sex with love. This is the one aspect of gay life that absolutely confounds me. I don't understand why gay relationships have to be so different from straight ones in this respect. Although sex is great, it should most definitely not be considered synonymous with love. Why do so many gay men believe, or want to believe, that they're the same thing?**
>
> **Anthony**

Dear Anthony,

Dissecting love has always provided people with an inexhaustible source of discussion. Infinite numbers of definitions exist. Psychologists, for example, sometimes divide love into different categories, such as the love between intimate partners, the love between parents and children, and the love between friends. Let's assume here that you are talking about the romantic type of love.

In my experience, love between gay men is no less complicated than love in the heterosexual world. It is hardly a secret that a considerable percentage of homosexual men enjoy high levels of sexual activity. So it seems logical to assume that guys who have high "turnover rates" with their partners are less likely to be interested in love. Not that they too aren't looking for Mr. Right in the long run, but play the odds and you're left with the likelihood that having sex with them will "just be sex."

I don't necessarily agree, though, that most gay men confuse sex with love. Are there guys out there who confuse acts of sex with romantic feelings? Sure. Some might feel that sex is the entryway to love, while others believe that, because you're having sex with someone, love is automatically involved. From what I've seen and heard, however, most guys are pretty grounded about the notion that sex is sex, and they do separate this from love. It all depends what's on your agenda. Do you want romantic sex or unemotional sex? I think most guys know what they want going into sex. They choose whether they want sexual play, with no romantic feelings and no emotional ties, or whether they are looking for sex in a potential long-term and emotionally binding relationship between two people.

Why does it seem that more gay men choose noncommittal sex? Who knows? It may be genetics. It may be conditioned into us. It might even be the male biological need to spread our seed. Whatever the reason, it's always important to make sure your agenda matches that of the person you're sleeping with. Otherwise, someone is going to be upset.

> **Dear Dr. Keith,**
>
> **I am a girl who identifies as straight, but I have had relationships in the past with women. Does this make me bisexual, even though I am really mostly attracted to men?**
>
> **Francesca**

Dear Francesca,

I have never been a big fan of labels. While they can effectively sum up some people's orientation, they often fail for others.

Calling yourself bisexual would tell people you're attracted to both men and women, but it doesn't indicate which you're more strongly attracted to. On the other hand, identifying yourself as heterosexual ignores any draw you might have towards women.

My advice is to be honest to others while staying true to yourself. Never compromise your integrity. Choose an identification only if you feel it fits you well and you want people to know that about you. If a label makes you uncomfortable, choose to not label yourself at all.

**❝ Dear Dr. Keith,**

**I'm over 50 years old, and I was wondering what the age limit is in Ontario for someone to be considered a minor. I have a 17-year-old friend who would like to have sex with me, but I certainly would not want to be charged for having sex with a minor. ❞**

**John**

Dear John,

Whether we agree or not, the legal age in Canada for most kinds of sex is 14. The exception is anal sex, for which the legal age is 18. That means you could legally have oral sex with your friend now, but not anal sex until he turns 18.

I urge you to be careful regardless. Your friend is very young, and his decision may not be well thought out. Keep in mind that he is at a very different stage in his life than you are in yours, which could cause problems for you both in the future. And, of course, there are many people who have strong convictions about such an age discrepancy. If others found out, you could stand to lose a lot.

However, I don't want to paint this with a solely negative brush. If your friend is truly mature enough to make a responsible decision, and you can avoid negative reactions from others, having sex could be a great experience for the two of you.

> **DID YOU KNOW**
> It is recorded that Julia the Elder (39 BC–AD 14), daughter of the Roman emperor Augustus, had sex with more than 80,000 people in her lifetime, both men and women. Her voracious sexual appetite was helped by the fact that she was stunningly beautiful. She was eventually exiled for her promiscuity.

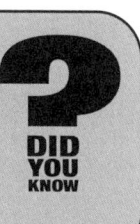

**❝ Dear Dr. Keith,**

**I am in an eighteen-year relationship. Things are getting pretty boring in the bedroom. How can I make them better? ❞**

**Roger**

Dear Roger,

Lack of passion in the bedroom as time passes is common for all couples, regardless of gender or sexual orientation. For some couples, it's not an issue. The love they have for each other remains, and their relationship takes a less sexual, or maybe even non-sexual, form.

But for those couples who want to keep their sexual intimacies enjoyable and exciting, here are some things to try. Get input from your partner beforehand so that you can decide exactly what would be interesting for both of you. No one should be uncomfortable or feel pressured. Besides, sitting down with your partner and playing "what if" scenarios might be very arousing in itself.

*Engage in role playing.* We all have fantasies about things we might find erotic and exciting under the right circumstances. For example, I have two friends who acted out a scene in which one was a mechanic and the other pulled up with his car to be "fixed." They said it was the best sex they ever had, right there on the garage floor.

*Avoid patterns.* Doing the same thing over and over leads to predictability, which for many is unappealing. Avoid the script; knowing exactly what you and your partner are going to do is a very efficient way of taking the fun out of sex. Change things around. Try using furniture, experimenting with new positions, using new toys. Even try changing your personality a bit (for example, become more aggressive or passive in the heat of the moment, if your partner is receptive to it).

*Change venues.* Avoid the bed. Try different rooms in the house; go to hotels; experiment with public places like washrooms or utility closets (just don't get caught!).

*Take a course.* In some cities, you can enrol in courses where they teach sexual techniques like oral sex.

*Use sexual aids.* Rent erotic films; try dildos, jock straps, or nipple clamps. Take a jaunt over to a local sex shop with your partner and buy something you both might like to try. Just make sure you read the instructions carefully and play safely.

Finally, go to your local GLBT bookstore or on-line for books with many more ideas. Getting ideas from friends never hurts, either.

Happy humping!

❝ **Dear Dr. Keith,**

**Can you explain "lesbian bed death"?** ❞

**Sam**

Dear Sam,

I hadn't heard this term before receiving a question about it on my TV show. I did some research on the Internet, and, to my surprise, references to "lesbian bed death" (LBD) are abundant there. The term seems to be used commonly in the lesbian community.

So what is it? In 1983, a book entitled *American Couples*, by Philip Blumstein and Pepper Schwartz, described lesbians as having less sex than either gay men or straight couples. This idea, seemingly confirmed by counsellors and other authorities, fuelled the notion that a lesbian couple in a long-term relationship will eventually lose interest in sex, being sexually intimate infrequently or not at all. The news spread through the lesbian community like wildfire. People of all backgrounds were talking about it, and some treated it as fact, even an inevitable tragedy.

The good news is that the existence of LBD is under extreme scrutiny, and many people dismiss it openly. There has never been clear evidence that a lesbian couple loses interest in sexual activity faster than any other type of couple. Losing interest in sex in a long-term relationship is certainly not unique to the lesbian bedroom. In my opinion, LBD is a myth created out of subconscious fear that as we age our enjoyment of sex will all be in the past.

If your love life is static or dwindling, there are many ways to heat things up. Don't claim defeat because of misinformation.

**DID YOU KNOW**

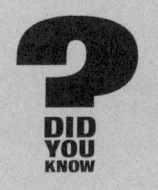

The "law of similarity" was a popular belief among ancient peoples. If a food resembled the genitalia, it was thought to be an aphrodisiac. Rhinocerous horns and oysters are two good examples, although neither has ever been proven to make you horny.

# Sources & Acknowledgements

I would like to briefly identify the sources I drew on for some of the "Did You Know" material:
- www.foothill.edu/clubs/gay-straight/faqs3.html
- www.psych.org/public_info/homose~1.cfm
- *Men's Health*, March 1996. Vol. 11, No. 2, p. 90.
- www.sexnewsdaily.com/issue/b463-092303.html
- www.sexualrecords.com/WSRtechnique.html
- www.sizes.com/people/penis.htm
- www.noharmm.org/snip.htm
- www.ozjokes.com
- www.caselaw.findlaw.com
- www.iglhrc.org
- www.sexualhealth.com
- www.obgyn.net/women/women.asp
- www.depts.washington.edu/wsstd/qa_frame.htm
- www.gender.org
- www.scarleteen.com

Two people were instrumental in helping me put this book together, and deserve mentioning:
- Michael Pickup, MD—thank you so much for helping me medically proof the manuscript. You've been an amazing friend as well—it's just too bad you're a surgeon. (Just kidding.)
- Laura Morris, RN—your much-needed assistance with the "girlie questions" is SO greatly appreciated. You are a fantastic resource

not only to your clients, but to the medical community at large. (And thanks for laughing at my reactions to some of your disturbing, yet enlightening, explanations. I'm having nightmares, by the way—the counselling bill is in the mail.)

I would also like to thank:

- Sherbourne Health Centre and Dr. Leslie Shanks, who directly and indirectly made accommodations allowing me to work on this project.
- Jason Hughes, Wendy Donnan, Dean Maher, and everyone working for Pridevision TV.
- Those at Whitecap Books who have been involved in the project, especially Robert McCullough, Barbara Pulling, Robin Rivers, Marial Shea and Jacqui Thomas. Thanks for taking a chance not only on a book like this, but also on a doctor with questionable writing skills. This has been a great experience.

# Index

## a
age of consent  *125-126*
anal pap smears  *93-94*
anal sex
  A-Spot  *61-62*
  Hepatitis A  *99-100*
  pain  *28-29*
  preparing for  *19, 27-28, 29-30*
anal warts. *See* Human Papilloma Virus
A-Spot  *61-62*

## b
bacterial vaginosis  *108-109, 112-113*
barebacking  *30-31*
bisexuality  *19-20, 95-96, 121-122, 124-125*
blow jobs. *See* oral sex
breast
  discharge  *104*
  tenderness  *54*
butt plugs  *35-36*
BV. *See* bacterial vaginosis

## c
cancer
  cervical  *99, 101-102*
  prostate  *75-76*

cancer, continued
  rectal  *93-94*
chafing  *73-74*
chlamydia  *84-86, 99*
clitoris  *51*
cock rings  *41-42*
condoms  *82-83*
  and vaginal irritation  *109-110*
crabs  *110-111*
cramps
  menstrual  *54-55, 103-104*
  muscle  *34-35*
cum. *See* semen

## d
dating services  *30-31*
discharge
  penile  *84*
  vaginal  *108-109, 102-103, 112-113*
doxycycline  *84-85*
douching
  anal  *27-28*
  vaginal  *28, 112-113*
dryness, vaginal  *53*

## e
ejaculate
  female  *51, 52*

**In 1886, a French woman was medically recorded to have 10 breasts.**

ejaculate, continued
    male  *41-42*
    *See also* semen
erections
    cock rings  *41*
    maintaining  *67-68*

**f**

family acceptance  *14*
fisting  *31-32, 32-34*
folliculitis  *89*

**g**

genital warts. *See* Human Papilloma Virus
gonorrhea  *83-84, 85-86, 99*
GLBT  *13-14*
G-Spot  *62*

**h**

Hepatitis A
    risk during menstruation  *103-104*
    in women  *99-100, 107-108*
Hepatitis B
    risk during menstruation  *103-104*
    in women  *99-100*
herpes simplex  *88-89, 89*
    and oral sex  *100-101*
    in women  *99-100*
HIV
    barebacking  *30-31*
    and "blow jobs"  *94-95*

HIV, continued
    breast milk  *104*
    disclosure  *90-91*
    and gonorrhea  *84-85*
    and herpes  *88-89*
    menstruation  *103-104*
    relationships  *93-94*
    in women  *99-100*
HPV. *See* Human Papilloma Virus
homosexuality, as an illness  *12-13, 23*
HSV. *See* Herpes Simplex
Human Immunodeficiency Virus. *See* HIV
Human Papilloma Virus
    anal  *86-88, 93-94*
    in women  *99, 101-102*

**l**

lesbian bed death  *128-129*
LGBT/LGBTTQI  *13-14*

**m**

marriage, same-sex  *20*
masturbation  *22-23*
    frequency  *39-40*
menstruation and arousal  *103-104*
monogamy  *16-17, 122-123*
muscle relaxants and anal sex  *28-29*

**n**

NGU. *See* non-gonococcal urethritis

---

**It is reported that the male members of the Walibri tribe of central Australia greet each other not by shaking hands but by shaking each others' penises.**

ASK DR. KEITH | 133

non-gonococcal urethritis *102-103*

**o**

oral sex *36-38*
  female *49-50*
  HIV *94-95*
  male *36-38*

**p**

pain
  anal *28-29, 39-40*
  testicular *72-73, 74-75*
  vaginal *49*
pap smears
  anal *93-94*
  cervical *101-102*
penis size *59-60*
PMS *54-55*
polygamy *16-17, 122-123*
premenstrual syndrome. *See* PMS
pussy fart *52*
prostate gland *41, 60-61, 62-63*

**r**

relationships
  cheating *121*
  gay vs. straight *119-120*
  male vs. female *16-17*
  moving in *120-121*
  sex and love *123-124*
  with straight persons *17-18*

relationships, continued
  *See also* monogamy, polygamy

**s**

semen
  blood *75-76*
  consistency *76-77*
  production and calories *41-42*
  seminal vesicles *41*
sex
  boredom *126-127*
  casual *15-16, 21-22*
  problems. *See* sexual dysfunction
  *See also* anal sex, oral sex
sexual dysfunction
  erectile *67-69, 69-70*
  orgasm *64-67*
sexual orientation, changing *12-13*
sexually transmitted diseases. *See* sexually transmitted infections
sexually transmitted infections
  and menstruation *103-104*
  and sexual orientation *94-95*
  swimming pools and hot tubs *81*
  in women *99-100*
  *See also* specific infections
staphylococcus *81-82*

**In fourteenth-century Europe, it was acceptable for noblemen to leave their genitals hanging out of their clothing in public.**

STDs. *See* sexually transmitted infections
STIs. *See* sexually transmitted infections
syphilis in women  *99*

**t**
testicles
  pain  *72-73*
  position  *71-72*
tongue piercing  *106-107*
toys
  cleaning  *109-110*
  cock rings  *40-42*
  dildos  *39-40*
  plugs  *35-36*

transgendered and transsexual  *18*
transvestite  *18*
trichomonas  *107*

**u**
urinary tract infections, recurrent  *105-106*

**v**
Viagra  *69-70*

**w**
warts. *See* Human Papilloma Virus, anal warts

**y**
yeast infections  *108-109, 109-110*

---

**Dr. John Harvey Kellogg was strongly against sexual gratification outside of marriage. He created "Corn Flakes" as a simple, nutritional breakfast to replace eating meat, which he felt caused people to masturbate and have sex with others. He also openly advocated circumcision without anesthetic, and the pouring of acid on women's genitals also to discourage sex.**

ASK DR. KEITH | 135

# About the Author

Born and raised in Fredericton, New Brunswick, Dr. Keith Loukes holds a Bachelor of Science degree in Bio-Psychology (UNB, 1996) and is a Doctor of Medicine (Memorial University, 2001). He completed a residency in Family Practice at the University of Toronto, where he was inspired to work with health issues particular to the lesbian, gay, bisexual and transsexual community, including HIV.

After finishing his residency, Dr. Keith was hired as an LGBT primary care physician by the Sherbourne Health Centre, a non-profit organization whose mandate is to offer health care to the LGBT community along with other under-serviced populations. Host of Pridevision TV's interactive health Q&A show, *By Appointment...*, Dr. Keith also appears in other media such as his "Health and the Weather" segment on *The Weather Network*, and has been interviewed in national publications such as *Outlooks* and *Eye*.

His favourite moment in medicine occurred in the middle of in-hospital emergency when he was mistaken for the janitor, handed a mop, and told by a nurse "you shouldn't wear a stethoscope, people might think you're a doctor."